Sign Languag

Sign Languages: Structures and Contexts provides a succinct summary of major findings in the linguistic study of natural sign languages. Focusing on American Sign Language (ASL), this book:

- offers a comprehensive introduction to the basic grammatical components of phonology, morphology, and syntax with examples and illustrations;
- demonstrates how sign languages are acquired by Deaf children with varying degrees of input during early development, including no input where children create a language of their own;
- discusses the contexts of sign languages, including how different varieties are formed and used, attitudes towards sign languages, and how language planning affects language use;
- is accompanied by e-resources, which host links to video clips.

Offering an engaging and accessible introduction to sign languages, this book is essential reading for students studying this topic for the first time with little or no background in linguistics.

Joseph C. Hill is Assistant Professor in the Department of American Sign Language and Interpreting Education at the National Technical Institutes for the Deaf in Rochester Institute of Technology, USA.

Diane C. Lillo-Martin is Board of Trustees Distinguished Professor of Linguistics at the University of Connecticut and a Senior Research Scientist at Haskins Laboratories, USA.

Sandra K. Wood is Assistant Professor of Linguistics and ASL Program Coordinator at the University of Southern Maine, USA.

Routledge Guides to Linguistics

Series Editor: Betty J. Birner is a professor of linguistics and cognitive science in the Department of English at Northern Illinois University.

Routledge Guides to Linguistics are a set of concise and accessible guidebooks, which provide an overview of the fundamental principles of a subject area in a jargon-free and undaunting format. Designed for students of linguistics who are approaching a particular topic for the first time, or students who are considering studying linguistics and are eager to find out more about it, these books will both introduce the essentials of a subject and provide an ideal springboard for further study.

This series is published in conjunction with the Linguistic Society of America (LSA). Founded in 1924 to advance the scientific study of language, the LSA plays a critical role in supporting and disseminating linguistic scholarship both to professional linguists and to the general public.

Is English Changing?
Steve Kleinedler

Why Study Linguistics
Kristin Denham and Anne Lobeck

Sign Languages
Structures and Contexts
Joseph C. Hill, Diane C. Lillo-Martin and Sandra K. Wood

More information about this series can be found at www.routledge.com/series/RGL

Sign Languages

Structures and Contexts

Joseph C. Hill,
Diane C. Lillo-Martin and
Sandra K. Wood

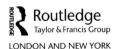
Routledge
Taylor & Francis Group
LONDON AND NEW YORK

Linguistic Society of America

First published 2019
by Routledge
2 Park Square, Milton Park, Abingdon, Oxon OX14 4RN

and by Routledge
52 Vanderbilt Avenue, New York, NY 10017

Routledge is an imprint of the Taylor & Francis Group, an informa business

© 2019 Joseph C. Hill, Diane C. Lillo-Martin and Sandra K. Wood

The right of Joseph C. Hill, Diane C. Lillo-Martin and Sandra K. Wood to be identified as authors of this work has been asserted by them in accordance with sections 77 and 78 of the Copyright, Designs and Patents Act 1988.

British Library Cataloguing-in-Publication Data
A catalogue record for this book is available from the British Library

Library of Congress Cataloging-in-Publication Data
Names: Hill, Joseph Christopher, author. | Lillo-Martin, Diane C. (Diane Carolyn), 1959– author. | Wood, Sandra K., author.
Title: Sign languages: structures and contexts / Joseph C. Hill, Diane C. Lillo-Martin and Sandra K. Wood.
Description: New York: Routledge, 2019. |
Series: Routledge guides to linguistics | Includes bibliographical references and index.
Identifiers: LCCN 2018038422| ISBN 9781138089167 (hardback) | ISBN 9781138089174 (pbk.) | ISBN 9780429020872 (e-book)
Subjects: LCSH: Sign language.
Classification: LCC HV2474 .H475 2019 | DDC 419—dc23
LC record available at https://lccn.loc.gov/2018038422

ISBN: 978-1-138-08916-7 (hbk)
ISBN: 978-1-138-08917-4 (pbk)
ISBN: 978-0-429-02087-2 (ebk)

Typeset in Times New Roman
by codeMantra

Visit the eResources: www.routledge.com/9781138089174

Contents

List of figures

List of tables

Acknowledgments

We would like to thank Betty Birner for inviting us to prepare this book, and for her comments on an earlier draft.

Most of the illustrations used in this book are taken from signs in the online lexical resource ASL Signbank (aslsignbank.haskins. yale.edu), which is licensed under a Creative Commons Attribution-NonCommercial-ShareAlike 4.0 International License. We are extremely grateful to Dr. Julie Hochgesang, the leader of the Signbank project, for her assistance, and to Carmelina Kennedy, who has helped in the production of very many Signbank entries and illustrations, including the ones used here. We also thank Doreen L. Simons for modelling some of the images used in Chapters 4 and 5.

We would like to thank Dr. Ceil Lucas for granting us the permission to use the video samples from her sociolinguistic projects: Sociolinguistic Variation in American Sign Language (BSC-9310116), Sociolinguistic Variation in American Sign Language, Phase II (BCS-9709522), and The Structure and History of Black American Sign Language (BCS-0818736). We recognize that her research team's projects mark important milestones in collecting representative samples of the American Deaf community with social- and geographic-based variation.

Research reported here was supported in part by the National Institute on Deafness and other Communication Disorders of the National Institutes of Health under Award Number R01DC013578. The content is solely the responsibility of the authors and does not necessarily represent the official views of the National Institutes of Health.

Chapter 1

Introduction

1.1 Sign languages and their users

Sign languages are produced by the hands, face, and body and perceived primarily visually, in contrast to spoken languages, which are produced by the mouth and vocal tract and perceived primarily auditorily (although manual gestures and visual perception of gestures and mouth movements are also important for spoken languages). Natural sign languages emerge (are not invented) when Deaf people form a community, often through educational systems. Sign languages are, therefore, primarily the languages of Deaf people, who cherish them for their cultural and community-building value.

It is important to recognize the connection between sign languages and Deaf communities. Until relatively recently, Deaf communities have been told (explicitly and implicitly) that their "sign communication" was inferior, broken, unimportant, or insufficient. Educational systems and the broader hearing majority community would stress the value of learning the spoken language, even at the expense of the sign language. In fact, such attitudes persist, both in areas where the national sign language has not been deeply studied linguistically and in areas where it has been studied but the focus for economic advancement is on the spoken language. However, the natural sign languages of Deaf communities are completely linguistic, rule-governed, capable of expressing anything, and fully worthwhile. We unreservedly endorse such affirmations of the value of sign languages and promote their use in all aspects of the lives of Deaf people.

Who belongs to the Deaf community? The "d" is capitalized to reinforce the view that Deaf communities form cultural groups with practices and values that are in some cases distinct from those of non-Deaf communities. These cultural effects are passed down within the community, from parents to children in some cases, but more often through interactions of Deaf people from different families. The leaders of Deaf communities are usually Deaf adults who were raised with Deaf parents or within the community from a very early age. Generally, members of the Deaf community are audiologically deaf or hard-of-hearing (and they shun the label "hearing impaired"). The hearing children born to Deaf parents are often known as Codas (from the name of an organization, CODA, 'children of Deaf adults'), and they are sometimes part of the Deaf community.

It is important to note that people have many identities with intersectional effects, and in this respect, not all Deaf people have the same experiences, values, and life view. A Deaf person's identity as Deaf will be affected by their identity in other ways, including race, ethnicity, gender identity, etc. Almost all research on the American Deaf community has focused only on a subset of Deaf people, so it is important to bear in mind that others might share some but not all of the characteristics described here.

Sign languages are, then, Deaf languages. Just as with the languages of other minority groups who have experienced oppression, hearing researchers who benefit from the study of sign languages (both in personal satisfaction and in economic, career, and other means) must acknowledge the primacy of Deaf signers and treat their language with the utmost respect.

1.2 Sign languages and American Sign Language

Sign languages can be studied and described as a group – sign languages in comparison to spoken languages (while some people prefer the term "signed" languages as a parallel to "spoken" languages, we use the term "sign languages"). It should be kept clearly in mind, however, that different sign languages are indeed different languages, contrary to those who might think that "sign language" is a single, uniform system used among Deaf communities all around the world. Therefore, any particular sign or phenomenon discussed here should be understood as part of a particular sign language. With this in mind, our focus in this book is on American Sign Language (ASL), the sign language used in the United States and most of Canada. Almost all the examples we discuss will come from ASL; in fact, they will generally come from a mainstream variety of ASL that is commonly used among relatively educated Deaf people, such as those who have attended Gallaudet University. We will discuss other varieties of ASL from time to time and focus on variation in Chapter 8.

Although our focus is on ASL, which is a distinct language from other sign languages, many of the grammatical phenomena we discuss have close analogues in other sign languages. There are several possible reasons for this. The first is historical relationships among sign languages. ASL emerged in the United States following the establishment of its first school for Deaf children, the American School for the Deaf (ASD), in Hartford, Connecticut in 1817. This school was the impetus for a community of Deaf people to gather together; when such a community is formed, a sign language emerges (see Chapter 8 for more information about the emergence and history of ASL). Prior to the establishment of the school, Deaf people may have used some "homesigns" (see Chapter 7), and some of them used Martha's Vineyard Sign Language, a "village sign language" that emerged among both Deaf and hearing people due to a high rate of deafness on Martha's Vineyard, a small island off the coast of Massachusetts. In addition to these signs used by some of the founding members of the Deaf community at ASD, there was a strong influence from French Sign Language (LSF), because the school was founded by an American, Thomas Hopkins Gallaudet, who brought a Deaf graduate from a Paris school for the Deaf, Laurent Clerc, who used LSF with the students. Thereby, ASL emerged as a language with LSF as one of its source languages, along with the signing used in various places of the United States. Because a number of schools in other countries were also founded around the same time by graduates from the school in Paris, there are many sign languages used in Europe and other places that have a historical connection to ASL.

When sign languages display common structural features, at times these may be due to a common historical connection to

LSF. However, there are some commonalities across sign languages that do not share this historical connection. This shows us that there may be linguistic characteristics associated with the manual/visual modality. The common ways that sign languages generally use space grammatically, in pronouns, verb agreement, and classifiers (see Chapter 3), may be among such characteristics. In addition, sign languages are able to take advantage of visual iconicity, to a greater degree than spoken languages are able to use iconicity in the auditory domain. This does not mean that sign languages are fully iconic, by any means, but there are some patterned similarities between visual referents and the ways that they are signed, which lead to certain similarities between different sign languages.

Given the observations that sign languages around the world are distinct, one might think that each sign language is a signed version of the spoken language used in its context – English for ASL, French for LSF, etc. This too is a misconception. Natural sign languages emerge in the contexts described as independent languages and have a grammar that is distinct from that of any nearby spoken languages. This is not to say that there is no relationship between a sign language and a surrounding spoken language; on the contrary, most sign language users are bilingual, at least to some extent, and as is typical in bilingual communities, each language can have some influence on the other. Nevertheless, the grammars are generally quite different, and there should be no expectation that the sign language works the way the spoken language does.

Here we are discussing the natural sign languages of Deaf communities. In an effort to educate Deaf children in the dominant spoken language, some people have invented sign systems to represent spoken languages manually. These systems, known in the United States as various forms of Signed English or Manually Coded English (MCE), are artificial and do not follow the same structural generalizations as ASL does. However, continuing exposure to MCE can also be a source of language influence, so that at least for some signers, certain properties of English may have been incorporated into their signing, just as a language may "borrow" words from another language. In general, we will aim to describe ASL as it is used by Deaf signers; when there are properties that are shared between ASL and English, whether by

accident or by borrowing, they will be discussed if they are suffi-
ciently integrated in the ASL used by native signers. It is not our
aim to discuss forms of Signed English, except in cases of explicit
contrast with ASL.

1.3 Key linguistic concepts

We have already used the term "grammar" several times. What do
we mean when we use this term? Within linguistics, "grammar"
refers to the unconscious mental rules that govern linguistic behavior. These rules are unconscious, but linguists have taken on
the task of trying to figure them out, based on the kinds of linguistic behaviors that speakers produce. This task can be compared
to the task of figuring out how a skilled rider controls and manipulates a bicycle by observing the rider – both as they successfully
maneuver hairpin turns and as some quirk causes them to lose
control. Although a cyclist may well have experienced explicit instruction, most of what they do is by instinct, as they figure out
the ways that leaning one way or putting pressure another will
keep them going. The researcher watches this and attempts to determine the physical and biological forces that combine to enable
this feat. While the analogy is not exact, linguists do observe various kinds of linguistic behavior (including ungrammaticalities)
and attempt to deduce the hidden rules that underlie the behavior.

It should be clear that these rules are "descriptive" – the
researcher is attempting to discover what patterns are present in the
behaviors observed. This is very different from the "prescriptive"
rules that "grammar teachers" or "grammar guides" espouse;
prescriptive rules are rules that are intended to inform a speaker
how to speak or write "properly." In our bicycle example, these
are the rules such as "signal well in advance of a turn" or "stay in
the bike lane." While there are some contexts in which such prescriptive rules may be useful, they are not the stuff of linguistics
and they are not our focus here. Descriptive rules are generally
not known explicitly, though linguists and speakers may develop
metalinguistic awareness of them, by thinking and talking about
language as the object of study.

In addition to focusing on descriptive rules, linguists attempt
to describe a speaker's competence, which is the knowledge of the

rules, rather than the actual performance at any particular time. Analyses are based on performance data, but linguists are also interested in abstract knowledge that assumes complete memory and processing capacity, just like physicists may study gravity in an environment free of friction. We do not, however, ignore context, and find that it is helpful to understand all the factors that affect performance in addition to the grammatical principles.

The rules of a mental grammar can be divided into several different domains. In this book, we will focus on the following three: phonology, morphology, and syntax. The rules of phonology are those rules that govern the pieces of words, or "sublexical units" (sub = beneath; lexical = word). For spoken languages, these are individual sounds that can be combined to make words. As is the custom in linguistics, when we talk about the sounds used we will write them within slash brackets, like /b/, /d/, and /g/. For sign languages, the sublexical units are not sounds, but there are pieces that combine to make a sign, including a handshape, a location, and a movement. We will discuss aspects of the phonology of ASL in Chapter 2. Note that a distinction can be made between phonology, the patterning of the pieces of words, and phonetics, a more precise characterization of the forms, how they are produced and perceived. While there is some interesting work on sign language phonetics, we will not discuss that domain in this book.

Morphology is the study of "morphemes," the minimal units of meaning. Some words, like "minimum," "unit," and "mean," have one morpheme; others, like "meaning," "units," and "minimize," have more than one. In addition to identifying the units, morphology studies how they are organized, such as how they combine to make new words, and how they are used within sentences. We will discuss ASL morphology in Chapter 3.

Syntax is the study of sentence structure. When different words combine to produce a sentence, the way they are organized is due to the relationship between syntax and meaning. One kind of organization will fit one kind of meaning, while a different organization will be interpreted in a different way. One kind of example to illustrate this crucial role of organization is *structural ambiguity*. Consider the sentence, "The woman messaged the man with a cell phone." The phrase "with a cell phone" can be interpreted as explaining how the message was sent by the woman; that is, it can modify the verb "messaged." Alternatively, it can modify the object "the man" if it is interpreted as his cell phone, or one that he is holding; the message could have been sent via a messenger rather than a text. Syntax helps to explain why sentences can have different interpretations by appealing to the idea of an abstract structure connecting the words. Similarly, different kinds of sentences can be used for different purposes, such as making a statement, denying something, or asking a question. The abstract structure of these different sentence types as used in ASL will be discussed in Chapter 4.

There are other aspects of grammar that will not be discussed much in this text, especially semantics, the study of meaning. Recently, there has been a lot of new research on sign language semantics, so this field is growing rapidly. Here, we will only touch on aspects of meaning as they relate to other areas of study.

In addition to components of grammar, this book will include discussions of other areas of sign linguistics, including developmental psycholinguistics (language acquisition) and sociolinguistics (language and society). Together, these chapters will give the reader an overview of the basics of ASL linguistics, and we hope they will inspire readers to learn more through additional sources.

1.4 Using this book

This text was written primarily for undergraduate students and others with an interest in sign language linguistics. We expect that most readers will have some knowledge of a sign language or some knowledge of linguistics, but we do not assume knowledge of either, in order to reach a broader audience. The ideal class using this text might be one with a mixture of signers and (budding) linguists, who can learn from each other and enhance the book's contents with other information.

Each chapter includes a set of "Discussion Questions," some of which we hope will cause readers to think deeply and speculate based on the information given. The chapters also include a brief annotated list called "Further reading," which we hope you will use to further your investigation of topics of interest. In addition, there is a more complete bibliography. We have avoided citing the sources for information within the text for the sake of readability.

We want to make clear that the findings we summarize are due to the work of a wide range of scholars, and by no means our own claims alone. Readers can use the reference lists as a springboard to further research on each topic.

In a number of places, we use a special font to illustrate the ASL handshapes we discuss in this book. It should be noted that sometimes the standard form of the handshape used in the font has to be modified in a real sign, such as when it is facing a different direction or slightly changed, which we will note in its description.

ASL has no established writing system. For this reason, linguistic works use glosses to represent signs. Glosses are English words written in all capitals that stand for signs. The English word is only to be used as a label for a sign, and generally the label that is chosen has some relationship to the sign, but the range of interpretations of the English word is not necessarily the same as that of the ASL sign. For example, the ASL sign MILK means essentially the same thing as the English word "milk," but the English word "run" includes a range of meanings that are not expressed by the ASL sign RUN. In addition, often there are variant signs that can be used to express the same meaning. In this case, an annotation (in lower case) is added to the gloss to specify which variant of a sign is intended.

Whenever possible, we use the glosses and annotations employed by the ASL Signbank (aslsignbank.haskins.yale.edu) and/ or ASL-LEX (asl-lex.org), two online lexical research resources for ASL. Because we have adopted the same glosses, readers can easily find and view video clips of individual signs on these sites, produced as citation forms without context. ASL Signbank is also the source for most of the still illustrations used in the book. It is important to keep in mind that still pictures cannot fully capture the appearance of a sign, although we do use photographic modifications to illustrate some aspects of the sign's movement. For example, the ASL sign for Signbank is shown in Figure 1.1. In the figure, the first part of the sign is shown as a more transparent image, while the second part is fully opaque. Check the homepage of ASL Signbank to see the sign in motion! Also, please see the Acknowledgments to this book and the "About" tab on the ASL Signbank site to read about conditions for use of the images and videos found on the site.

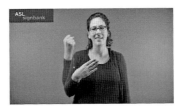

Figure 1.1   The sign for ASL Signbank: NS(ASB). Image: ASL Signbank, 2018.

The website to accompany this text (www.routledge.com/9781 138089174) contains examples of some of the signed utterances and phenomena that are discussed in the book, as well as other information (Table 1.1).

Table 1.1   Annotation Conventions

SIGN	Signs are written using glosses in upper case. The glosses are those used by ASL Signbank whenever possible. Glosses are words that stand for signs, but the signs have their own lexical, phonological, grammatical, and semantic properties.
SIGN-SIGN	When multiple words are written with a hyphen between them, it means that more than one English word is needed, but the gloss still stands for a single sign.
SIGNtag	A lower-case tag on an English gloss indicates which variant is intended.
DS_x(y)	DS stands for "depicting sign," also known as classifiers (see Section 3.5). The label DS is followed by a symbol indicating the handshape (which can be found in Signbank); the material in parentheses describes the sign.
IX(ref), IX_I	IX refers to an indexical pointing sign. The referent being pointed at can be indicated within parentheses following IX. IX_I is a point to the self.
nm SIGN SIGN	A line above a sign or signs indicates that a particular nonmanual marker is produced simultaneously with the signs. "br" stands for brow raise, "bf" stands for brow furrow, "hn" stands for head nod, and "hs" stands for head shake.
SIGN[+]	The [+] sign following a gloss indicates that the sign is reduplicated (repeated).

Further reading

Baker, A., van den Bogaerde, B., Pfau, R., & Schermer, T. (2016). *The linguistics of sign languages: an introduction.* Amsterdam, the Netherlands: John Benjamins Publishing Company.

This book goes in to more detail on many topics of sign linguistics, with examples from numerous sign languages, especially those in Europe. It does assume knowledge of basic linguistics.

Lane, H. (1984). *When the mind hears: a history of the deaf.* New York, NY: Random House.

This book is a thorough and interesting report of the history of the Deaf community, including the ways that sign languages have been an integral part of this.

Leigh, I. W., Andrews, J. F., & Harris, R. (2015). *Deaf culture: exploring deaf communities in the United States.* San Diego, CA: Plural Publishing, Inc.

This book provides a comprehensive coverage of Deaf culture with theoretical and practical information in education, psychology, cultural studies, technology, and the arts.

Pfau, R., Steinbach, M., & Woll, B. (Eds.). (2012). *Sign language – an international handbook.* Berlin, Germany: Walter de Gruyter.

This handbook discusses many aspects of sign language linguistics, with examples from sign languages around the world. It covers a wide range of topics but does assume some knowledge of linguistics.

Sandler, W., & Lillo-Martin, D. (2006). *Sign language and linguistic universals.* Cambridge, England: Cambridge University Press.

This book is an extensive dive into sign language grammar, especially morphology, phonology, and syntax. It assumes advanced knowledge of linguistic theory.

Valli, C., Lucas, C., Mulrooney, K., & Rankin, M. N. P. (2000). *Linguistics of American Sign Language.* Washington, DC: Gallaudet University Press.

This book includes overviews of ASL grammatical phenomena, exercises, and supplementary readings. It presupposes advanced knowledge of ASL.

Bibliography

Emmorey, K. (2002). *Language, cognition, and the brain: insights from sign language research.* Mahwah, NJ: Lawrence Erlbaum Associates.

Emmorey, K., & Lane, H. (Eds.). (2000). *The signs of language revisited*. Mahwah, NJ: Lawrence Erlbaum Associates.

Hochgesang, J. A., Crasborn, O., & Lillo-Martin, D. (2018). *ASL Signbank*. New Haven, CT: Haskins Laboratories, Yale University. https://aslsignbank.haskins.yale.edu

Klima, E. S., & Bellugi, U. (1979). *The signs of language*. Cambridge, MA: Harvard University Press.

Lane, H. (1989). *When the mind hears: a history of the deaf*. New York, NY: Random House.

Lane, H., & Philip, F. (1984). *The deaf experience: classics in language and education*. Cambridge, MA: Harvard University Press.

Meier, R. P., Cormier, K., & Quinto-Pozos, D. (Eds.). (2002). *Modality and structure in signed and spoken languages*. Cambridge, England: Cambridge University Press.

Stokoe, W. C. (1960). Sign language structure: an outline of the visual communication systems of the American deaf. In *Studies in linguistics: occasional papers*. Buffalo, NY: University of Buffalo.

Chapter 2

Phonology

This chapter begins the section of the book on grammar. Although many people think the word "grammar" refers to sentence structure, or worse, to prescriptive rules, it is actually a term to cover all of the unconscious rules that a person follows when they know a language (see also Chapter 1 for discussion of key concepts). We start the section by discussing the organization of linguistic units that are smaller than a word, that is, phonology. In the subsequent two chapters, we will discuss morphology, the ways that words are modified, and syntax, the formation of sentences. In each case, we will focus on how sign languages are similar to spoken languages, and we will point out important differences.

2.1 What is phonology?

Phonology is often described as the study of the sounds of language and their organization. If that is the way to look at phonology, it would be appropriate to say that sign languages do not have phonology. However, phonology is actually more abstract. It is about the ways in which words are made up of pieces that are not meaningful. It is about what these pieces are and how they work together. In spoken languages, the actual sounds that make up words are part of the study of phonology; yet, phonology is more concerned with the ways we can define these component pieces, how they change in different contexts (e.g., different words), and how they are organized.

With this in mind, we can begin to talk about phonology in sign languages. If there are component pieces that make up individual signs, then there is sign phonology. If there are implicit rules about the ways that the pieces can and cannot combine, then there is phonology. Indeed, one of the first linguistic discoveries about American Sign Language (ASL) is that "signs have parts" – that the components of individual signs can be identified and described, and that there are ways in which they combine and ways in which they do not combine (that is, constraints). In the following sections of this chapter, we will outline these component parts, explain some of the constraints on their combinations, and show that while sign languages display more simultaneity than spoken languages do, linearity is also important. Then, we will discuss "prosody" in sign languages – this is the area of phonology that connects to syntax, including rhythm and intonation. Finally, we will address the question of whether sign languages have the equivalent of syllables, which can be considered one of the fundamental organizing units of phonology.

2.2 Signs have parts

Consider a spoken word like "boat." If we break it down to the pieces of the spoken word, there are three units: /b/, /o/, and /t/ (the sounds are written within slashes to indicate that we mean sounds, not written letters; notice that sometimes two written letters are used to indicate one single sound). Although there is some correspondence between the sounds and the letters used to write them, they should not be confused. English spelling is famous for not making a one-to-one correspondence between letters and sounds. When we study phonology, we ignore the written form and concentrate on how the word is actually pronounced. Therefore, if we compare the pronunciation of "boat" with the pronunciation of "boot," we find that the only difference is in the vowel; "boot" uses the vowel sound /u/. "Boat" and "boot" are a minimal pair – two words that are pronounced the same except for one sound, in this case, the vowel. Likewise, "boat" and "coat" are a minimal pair – they are the same except for the first sound, which is /b/ in "boat" and /k/ in "coat."

Similarly, we can consider the production of a sign by breaking it down into its component parts, and we can compare signs that

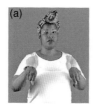 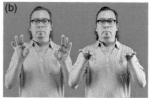

Figure 2.1 Minimal pair in ASL: (a) POSSIBLE and (b) DYE. Images: ASL Signbank, 2018.

are minimal pairs. Consider the sign POSSIBLE,[1] illustrated in Figure 2.1a. The sign is produced using both hands in a fist handshape (✊), in front of the signer in neutral space with palms facing forward; the sign movement involves repeated movement at the wrist so that the palm faces down. The sign DYE, illustrated in Figure 2.1b, is minimally different; it uses a different handshape (🖐) but is produced in the same location and with the same movement.

Because the signs POSSIBLE and DYE are a minimal pair, we can see that the ✊ handshape and the 🖐 handshape are distinctive phonological units, parallel to the /b/ vs. /k/ in "boat" and "coat." More generally, the configuration of the hands is one of the significant phonological units in sign languages (by "configuration" we mean the way the hand is formed by having certain fingers extended, curved, or lax, other fingers closed, and similar features). Similar comparisons can be drawn to show that the location of a sign (neutral space in front of the signer in these examples), and the movement (bending at the wrist) are phonological units. Most phonological analyses of sign languages are based primarily on identifying signs by giving information about their handshape, location, and movement. These components are sometimes called "parameters."

Additional information is needed for a full description of signs, so that some researchers propose that there are two more parameters in addition to handshape, location, and movement. First, there is the orientation of the palm. Often, this is determined by the other parameters, but sometimes orientation can be independently manipulated and even lead to minimal pairs. For example, the signs CHILDREN and THING (shown in

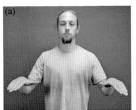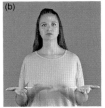

Figure 2.2 Minimal pair differing only in palm orientation: (a) CHILDREN and (b) THING. Images: ASL Signbank, 2018.

Figure 2.2) both involve a flat palm handshape, produced in the space immediately in front of the signer's waist level, with a movement that uses small bounces toward the side. In CHILDREN, the palm of the hand is facing downward, while in THING, the palm is facing upward. This minimal pair indicates that differences in orientation can be distinctive, which is why it can be considered a parameter. However, there are very few minimal pairs involving orientation and it is usually predictable, which is why it is often considered a minor parameter.

The proposed fifth parameter is facial expression (or nonmanual marking). So far, we have concentrated on what the hands are doing when we describe signs, and most of the time attention is on this manual component. However, some signs are also produced with a specific nonmanual component. For example, the sign ACCOMPLISH is usually produced along with a mouth movement that involves starting from closed lips and suddenly opening the mouth while the sign is produced. The expression is called "pah" because the mouth moves similarly to the way that it would move when pronouncing that syllable. A few signs like ACCOMPLISH typically are produced with a very specific nonmanual component – in order to say the sign properly, the nonmanual part must be included. For these signs, the nonmanual component can constitute a fifth parameter.

Note that nonmanual marking is used in many different ways, including as a way to indicate sentence types such as questions and negation (see Chapter 4). Nonmanual markers serving different functions can even be combined, such as when a person might ask whether or not the other had success (for example, on an exam). Then, the "pah" marker for ACCOMPLISH would combine with the yes/no question marker (which includes raising the eyebrows and tilting the head). We will discuss nonmanual marking in more detail in Section 2.5.

If signs can usually be described by giving their handshape, location, and movement, does this mean that we will be able to list all possible signs once we combine every possible handshape with every possible location and movement? Combining a possible handshape with any possible location and any possible movement could give us candidate signs, but not always a legal sign. Compare the English examples "boat" and "coat" again. We know that English words can make use of the sounds /b/, /k/, /o/, and /t/ – so can we make a word /bkot/? Or /tbo/? Or /otk/? Even though these "candidate" words are made up of possible pieces, they are not possible words. They can be contrasted with /bok/, which could be a word of English. The difference between possible words that don't happen to be part of the language, and impossible combinations of phonological elements, can be accounted for by considering constraints on signs, which we turn to next.

2.3 Signs are constrained

The sign APPLEx is made by using a fist-like handshape placed at the side of the mouth using a twisting movement. If we know that the side of the eye is another possible place for a sign, what happens if we use the same fist-like handshape with a twisting movement there? The result is a real sign, ONION. What about the contralateral side of the chest (the side opposite to the signing hand), which is the location used for signs like POLICE? Even though all the pieces are legitimate, there is no ASL sign made by using the same fist-like handshape and twisting movement on the contralateral chest position. But this is probably an "accidental gap" – there could be a sign made like that, and perhaps someday there will be. On the other hand, there are many possible combinations of sign phonological elements whose outcome would not be considered a possible sign. What restricts these combinations?

Several constraints have been proposed to account for some of the patterns seen in signs (there are likely additional constraints, but here we focus on three). These constraints apply to monomorphemic signs – this means the signs are not made by combining meaningful parts, but are themselves a single morpheme (see Chapter 3 for further discussion of morphemes). The first we will discuss is a constraint on the ways that handshape can change during a sign. The other two are constraints on two-handed signs.

The signs we have discussed so far have only one handshape, but there are many signs that use a change in handshape, such as the signs UNDERSTAND and PICK, illustrated in Figure 2.3. In UNDERSTAND, the handshape changes from 👆 to 👆; in PICK, the handshape changes from 👆 to 👆. If we have to specify that some signs have two handshapes, can a sign have any two handshapes at all?

The fact is that ASL signs do not arbitrarily combine different handshapes; instead, there is a strict constraint on the way that different handshapes can be used. This constraint is based on the observation that each handshape involves a set of selected fingers, with the other fingers unselected. Sometimes the selected fingers are extended, with the unselected fingers closed, as in the handshapes 👆, 👆, 👆, 👆, etc. In other cases, the selected fingers are closed, with the unselected fingers extended, as in the handshape 👆. In 👆, the index finger (selected) touches the thumb, while the middle, ring, and pinky fingers are extended. Now, we can introduce the constraint as follows:

Selected Fingers Constraint
Only one group of fingers may be selected in a morpheme.

Let's see how this constraint works. If the index finger is selected, it can be extended while the other fingers are closed, as in the

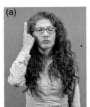
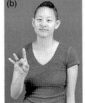

Figure 2.3 ASL signs with more than one handshape: (a) UNDER-STAND and (b) PICK. Images: ASL Signbank, 2018.

handshape 🖐. Then, the selected index finger can bend, in a sign like BIRD, or it can curve, in a sign like ASKonex. It's even possible for the selected finger to start closed and open up to a 🖐 handshape, as in UNDERSTAND. But no sign starts with the index finger selected (say, extended) and changes to the pinky selected (extended), as would be obtained if a handshape change went from 🖐 to 🖐.

In SUBMIT, all the fingers are selected, but they start closed, in a fist; because of the handshape change, they all end up extended. In PICK, the middle finger is selected; the unselected fingers are extended throughout the sign, while the selected finger starts extended and changes to closed, touching the thumb.

It's important to remember that you can't always tell which fingers are selected by looking at which are extended, and the selected fingers may be visible in the first handshape or in the second. Just pay attention to which fingers change their position in a sign – those are the selected fingers; the others stay in the same configuration throughout the sign, as they are unselected.

Now we will turn to look at two other constraints; they refer to two additional phonological notions we need to explain: handedness and markedness.

Handedness refers to the ways the two hands work together to form a sign. Many hands are produced with only one hand. However, there are also signs produced with both hands. While the two hands are physically independent, they must work together in one of two ways when forming a single sign. These ways are characterized by the two constraints.

Markedness is a pervasive concept in linguistics. Put simply, many components of grammar will have marked and unmarked possibilities. The unmarked option is easier to produce, more common within the language, more common across languages, and/or easier to learn. The marked option is harder to produce/learn, and used in more restricted contexts.

Now, we are ready for the two constraints. These constraints apply to two-handed signs that are monomorphemic.

Symmetry Constraint
If both hands of a two-handed sign move independently, then they must be specified for the same location, the same

handshape, the same movement (simultaneously or alternating), and the orientation must be symmetrical or identical.

Dominance Constraint
If the hands of a two-handed sign do not share the same handshape, then one hand must be passive while the active hand articulates the movement, and the passive hand must use an unmarked handshape (⬆, ⬆, ⬆, ⬆, ⬆, ⬆, ⬆).

Let's see what the constraints allow and prohibit.

First, the constraints have nothing to say about one-handed signs. There are surely additional constraints on possible combinations of handshape, movement, and location within one-handed signs, but those constraints are separate from the Symmetry and Dominance constraints.

Many two-handed signs are of the type determined by the Symmetry constraint. For example, the ASL sign THRILL, illustrated in Figure 2.4a, is a two-handed sign in which the hands have the same location (chest), the same handshape (open-⬆), the same movement (simultaneous movement up and arcing to the side), and the same orientation (palm toward the signer). An example of a symmetrical sign with alternating movement is ASL EXPLANATION, illustrated in Figure 2.4b. In this sign, the two hands produce their movement alternately, using the same handshapes, locations, and orientations.

Signs like BUTTER, illustrated in Figure 2.4c, are subject to the Dominance condition. Note that signers may differ in whether their dominant hand for signing is their right hand or their left hand; the descriptions given here will refer to dominant and nondominant hand without usually referring to which is right or left. In BUTTER, notice that the two hands do not share the same handshape: the dominant hand uses the ⬆ handshape, while the nondominant hand uses the ⬆ handshape. The nondominant hand is passive while the dominant hand performs the action, which involves moving the fingers of the dominant hand across the bottom part of the open palm of the nondominant hand. As the Dominance constraint requires, the nondominant hand uses one of the unmarked handshapes (⬆).

Finally, there are two-handed signs which are not subject to either the Symmetry constraint or the Dominance constraint,

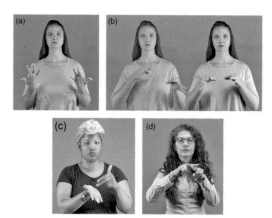

Figure 2.4 Types of signs based on handedness: (a) THRILL, two-handed symmetrical (simultaneous); (b) EXPLANATION, two-handed symmetrical (alternating); (c) BUTTER, two-handed sign subject to the Dominance condition; and (d) TRAIN, two-handed sign not subject to Symmetry or Dominance conditions. Images: ASL Signbank, 2018.

such as the sign TRAIN shown in Figure 2.4d. The Symmetry constraint applies if both hands move independently, but in this example, the nondominant hand is passive. The Dominance constraint applies if the two hands do not share the same handshape, but in TRAIN, both hands use the same handshape (🤏). Thus, signs made with one active hand acting on a passive hand, where both have the same handshape, are freely allowed (as long as other constraints, not specified here, are not violated).

There are some signs that violate the Symmetry or Dominance condition, but these conditions are respected by the majority of ASL signs. Sometimes the exceptions have a clear explanation, such as a sign that is borrowed from another sign language, or modified from an older form. These constraints appear to be generally active across natural sign languages. One of the criticisms of invented sign systems is that they often include signs that do not adhere to these constraints, since the people inventing these systems did not take into consideration the unconscious rules of natural sign languages.

2.4 Linearity and simultaneity

When the pieces of a spoken word combine, such as /b/, /o/, and /t/, they form a sequence: /bot/. In fact, if one inspects a graphical display of the acoustic event that makes a spoken word (called a sound spectrogram), it is not possible to make a sharp cut between the sounds – in our example, the /b/ is influenced by the /o/ and overlaps with it, and the /o/ overlaps with the /t/. Nevertheless, linearity plays a large role in spoken language phonology.

On the contrary, when the handshape, location, and movement of a sign combine, they are simultaneously produced. There is no movement without a handshape in a location – they all seem to combine at the same time. In the early days of sign language research, this simultaneity was the focus. However, researchers soon detected several ways in which linearity plays an important role. We will discuss some of these here, and come back to aspects of simultaneity in both sign languages and spoken languages in Section 2.5.

In signing a sentence, one sign follows the other (see also Chapter 4). This already shows that linearity plays a role in sign languages. But what about individual signs? Consider a sign like COMMITTEE, illustrated in Figure 2.5a. This sign is made with the ✐ handshape moving from the contralateral side of the chest to the ipsilateral side. The sign CHRISTIAN, illustrated in Figure 2.5b, has the same starting position and handshape, but it moves to a position on the ipsilateral waist. The fact that these two signs are different only in their second position shows that even within a sign, linearity or sequentiality can be important.

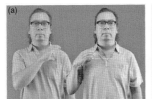

Figure 2.5 Signs differing in the second point of contact: (a) COMMITTEE and (b) CHRISTIAN. Images: ASL Signbank, 2018.

What about other signs? Consider the signs illustrated in Figures 2.3 and 2.4. Even if it's natural to think of these signs as having a simultaneous combination of handshape, location, and movement, it is also possible to break them down into sequences. For example, THRILL begins with the middle finger of each hand touching the chest and ends with the hands in neutral space. It can be described as having an initial location, and a movement toward a final location. The same handshape is used throughout the sign. This kind of arrangement can be notated as follows, where "L" stands for a location, "M" stands for a path movement, and "H" stands for a handshape. The linear order of the Ls and Ms indicates a temporal sequence. Putting the H on top and connecting it with lines to each L and M unit indicates that the same handshape is used with each L and M.

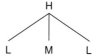

The sign STAND-UP uses a different type of structure. It is produced with the index and middle fingers of the dominant hand touching the palm of the nondominant hand. This is what the sign looks like at the end; the signer gets to that configuration by moving the dominant hand toward the nondominant hand. The beginning location is irrelevant. Therefore, this sign can be described as M L, missing any specific initial L, as shown below.

There are various reasons to think that it is important to specify the linearity of individual signs. We have already seen that some signs use a handshape change. To fully specify how these signs work, it is useful to talk about the initial handshape and the final handshape as linear notions. Also, let's consider how handshape change combines with path movement by looking at the sign THROW. The sign uses the index and middle fingers as selected, and it starts with the selected and unselected fingers closed into a fist. The sign begins near the signer's body. As the sign moves away from the body, the two selected fingers extend from the fist, so that the sign ends with the 𝄐 handshape. The movement of the fingers goes along with the path movement from close to the body to away from the body. Then, we can specify the beginning and ending locations with their handshapes, and we can say that the movement forms a transition between the handshapes while the path is traversed.

In Chapter 3, when we discuss sign morphology, we will see additional reasons to talk about the linear order within individual signs. It is clear that even individual signs may have a sequence, just like spoken words are composed of sounds in a sequence. However, it is true that signs have much more simultaneity than spoken words do. This is an effect of the modality – the large articulators with many subcomponents (arms, hands, fingers) of sign languages can combine elements in ways that the vocal articulators cannot. However, this is not to say that there is no simultaneous production of different elements even in spoken languages. They display a lot of simultaneity in the use of prosody, timing, rhythm, stress, and melody of speech. Is there anything like prosody in sign languages?

2.5 Sign language prosody

Prosody contributes a lot to how a language "sounds" – it provides rhythm and intonation, turning declarative sentences into questions and putting the emPHAsis on the right syLLAble. In spoken languages, there are three primary effects of prosodic organization: timing, stress, and pitch. Timing has to do with the slight pauses or holds that often (though not always) are marked with a comma or a period in written texts (for example, there may be a pause and even a breath between "Hello" and "my name is Lee"). Stress can be used to separate nouns from verbs (for example, the noun "protest" has stress on the first syllable (PROtest), while the verb "protest" has stress on the second syllable (proTEST)). Stress is also used for emphasis, or correction (as in, "No, I want the GREEN cup"). Intonation is the melody of a sentence; it is due to intonation that we can ask a question without changing anything else about a sentence (as in, "You're going to the show?").

Sign languages also have prosody, with some very sign-specific components. Timing is the most comparable to spoken language: there may be brief pauses or holds between sentences or phrases. Stress is used for emphasis like it is in speech; in ASL, stress is marked by the use of faster movement, tensed muscles, and sometimes larger movement or a change in the number of repetitions of a sign.

The most interesting (and modality-specific) case is the way that intonation is conveyed in sign languages: through nonmanual markers. Nonmanual markers are used, for example, to convey questions: the brows are raised and the head is tilted forward to indicate a polar question (polar questions, also known as yes/no questions, seek a response of "yes" or "no"); the brows are furrowed and the head might be tilted back to indicate a content question (content questions, also known as wh-questions, seek some kind of information in response; they will be discussed more in Chapter 4). It is important to understand the role of nonmanual markers in sign languages. Sometimes when nonsigners see people signing, they think the signer is very emotive because of the "exaggerated" use of facial expressions. But facial expressions are part of the nonmanual markers that contribute to sign language prosody. They are grammatical elements, just as the rising intonation to mark yes/no questions in many languages are part of the grammar of those languages. Vocal pitch is used to indicate a number of things, including emotions, but those aspects that are used to mark grammatical structures are part of the grammar. The same can be said for facial expressions and other nonmanuals: they can be used to indicate emotions, but they are also used in rule-governed, grammatical ways.

If nonmanual markers can be used grammatically, why are they considered to be a part of prosody? Prosody is the domain of language that expresses aspects of the grammar and the function of a linguistic unit through "suprasegmentals" – pieces of the utterance that are not associated with only one unit (one sound or one word), but spread over a domain (for example, a sentence). Rising intonation can spread over a short sentence, such as, "you going?", or a long sentence, such as "you going to the meeting in the auditorium at nine o'clock?". Similarly, the raised brows of a yes/no question spread over the full extent of the question, whether it contains one sign or many.

Researchers are still working to understand the full extent of sign language prosody. Furthermore, while it is clear that some nonmanual markers are part of prosody, it is also the case that there are many different types of nonmanual markers and they do not all behave in the same way. That is why nonmanual markers will come up in different sections of this book, since different markers will be discussed in the relevant contexts.

2.6 Are there syllables in sign languages?

The syllable is an important organizing unit in spoken languages. Many phonological processes apply based on where a sound is in a syllable; for example, constraints permit certain consonant clusters in syllable-initial position and others in syllable-final position, or sound changes may affect only syllable-initial or syllable-final sounds. Syllables are also important for metalinguistic phenomena such as poetry and literacy. Furthermore, this knowledge emerges relatively early; children begin learning to play with language at a young age, and clapping along with each syllable is one very early form of such play. In addition, syllables are timing units that play a role in language production and perception; we notice syllable-sized pieces most readily when we are processing language.

Is there an analogue to the syllable in sign languages? In order to answer this question in the affirmative, we need to see whether there are units that are based on phonological structure and do not correspond completely with a segment, a morpheme, or a word, yet play a role in sign languages. Such investigation has identified a syllable unit in sign languages.

Recall that in the discussion of linearity, we characterized a typical sign as having a sequence of a location, movement, location, with the same handshape throughout, using the structure repeated below. This is a typical signed syllable.

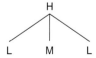

Most signs in ASL (and other sign languages) are monomorphemic words – that is, a single signed word contains only one morpheme (recall that a morpheme can roughly be described as a meaning-bearing unit). From what we've just written, it can be concluded that most monomorphemic signs are also monosyllabic – they have the L M L structure that corresponds to a single syllable. Are there monomorphemic words that have more than one syllable? Yes, there are several types. One example is the ASL sign APPOINTMENT, illustrated in Figure 2.6a. This sign has two M units. First, the dominant hand makes a quick circle above the nondominant wrist, while the handshape changes from open to closed (✊). Then, the hand moves straight downward to contact the wrist. In order to describe this, two movement units are needed: one for the circular movement and the other for the movement straight down. Each of these movement units is the core part of a syllable. Another example is MAGIC, illustrated in Figure 2.6b. This sign also has two syllables; it has a handshape change (closing) during the first syllable with circular movement, and another handshape change (opening) during the second syllable with path movement away from the signer (note that there are different versions of the sign MAGIC; this description applies to only one of them).

The syllable as just described is a timing unit, as can be detected by looking at the rhythm of signing; it is also a phonological unit, as we can see from the following constraint that applies to syllables. We have already introduced three constraints that apply to a morpheme (the Selected Fingers constraint, the Symmetry constraint, and the Dominance constraint). We now introduce a constraint on syllables:

Syllable-Level Hand Configuration Constraint
A syllable can contain at most two hand configurations.

 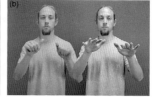

Figure 2.6 Signs with more than one syllable: (a) APPOINTMENT and (b) MAGIC. Images: ASL Signbank, 2018.

We know that signs can change their hand configuration, as we saw in the examples in Figure 2.3. However, such a change can take place at most once per syllable. The example MAGIC shows that this constraint applies to syllables, not morphemes (or words). In MAGIC, there is one handshape change during each syllable. If the constraint on handshape changes applied to morphemes, this kind of sign would not be allowed, since it is only one morpheme. However, it does have two syllables, which match the number of handshape changes.

As the examples discussed here illustrate, syllables are the units for the timing of handshape changes. When a handshape changes during a syllable, the change takes place over the full course of the syllable, not all at once at the beginning or end.

Are there other types of syllables in sign languages? Yes, there must be, since not all signs have the L M L structure. Signs always have some kind of movement in them; but while sometimes it is a path movement, symbolized as M, at other times it is "hand-internal" movement, such as wiggling the fingers, as in the sign SWELL illustrated in Figure 2.7a, or rapidly repeating bending of the fingers, as in the sign RABBIT-EARS illustrated in Figure 2.7b. Other signs involve a handshape change without path movement, as in UNDER-STAND, illustrated in Figure 2.3a. These kinds of movements are sufficient to make a signed syllable, but they are actually considered to be part of a sign that consists of only an L segment, since there is no path movement. They are symbolized as follows:

H
|
L

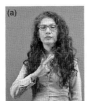

Figure 2.7 Signs with hand-internal movement only: (a) SWELL and (b) RABBIT-EARS. Images: ASL Signbank, 2018.

The H symbol stands for the handshape; in a full specification of the sign, the handshape change or "internal" movement would be marked on the H. Only one L is needed since the sign is made in only one place.

2.7 Conclusion

In this chapter, we have presented evidence for the phonological structure of signs. It was an initial analysis of sign phonology that jumpstarted linguistic approaches to sign languages, in the publication of the first dictionary of ASL that used a componential analysis of signs, led by William Stokoe with two Deaf colleagues in 1965. That analysis initiated the description of signs using information about handshape, location, and movement. Although Stokoe proposed new terminology and his notation system did not persist, his observation that signs are not holistic gestures but composed of meaningless parts has endured, and led the way for further research and recognition of sign languages.

As we have shown, not only are the component pieces of signs recognizable and analyzable, but they combine in linguistically rule-governed ways. Not every possible manual gesture is a possible sign, since constraints on the combination of pieces will rule out many feasible gestures. Understanding these constraints takes us a step further into understanding the nature of sign language phonology. There are many more detailed studies of sign formation that have motivated competing models, each attempting to account for the patterns in signs in a logical and elegant way.

We also reviewed the ways that signs have analogues to two important aspects of spoken language phonology: prosody and a syllabic unit of organization. We look for such analogues not because of any primacy of the phenomena in spoken languages, but only because findings about generalizations that hold for speech should be tested in sign languages. Linguists are interested in knowing what aspects of language structure are common across languages and which are specific to a particular type of language. As it turns out, prosody and syllables are not dependent on the spoken modality, but occur in sign languages as well.

This is not to say that there are no phonological differences of interest between sign languages and spoken languages. Clearly, there are many differences in the ways that signs and spoken words are formed, the most immediately obvious of which are the primary use of the hands versus the vocal tract. There is another important difference, which we have mentioned: although there is linearity in sign languages and there are multisyllabic words, the organization of signs is much more simultaneous than that of spoken words, and the vast majority of individual signed words are monosyllabic. These differences are clearly due to aspects of the visual-spatial modality; the relatively slower movement of the primary articulators over a much larger physical domain – and the perceptual advantages of such size – leads to a longer timing unit which packs a lot more information into it.

There are some ways in which these modality differences also lead to differences in the domains of morphology and syntax, which we will turn to next. We will also see, in Chapters 5–7, how these differences are acquired by early and late learners; and we will see, in Chapters 8–10, how they factor into differences across linguistic subgroups. Despite the persistent importance of modality differences, however, the strongest effect is a powerful deep similarity across languages of all types, demanding an equal degree of respect and esteem.

Discussion questions

1   What are the meaningless units that make up a sign?
2   What are minimal pairs like in sign languages compared to spoken languages?
3   Make up an illegal sign that violates the Selected Fingers constraint, one that violates the Symmetry constraint, and one that violates the Dominance constraint. Do you know any real signs that violate these constraints? Why do you think there might be signs that do not conform – what is it about these signs that allows them to be different?
4   Why is it important to ask whether sign languages have syllables? Would sign languages be somehow lesser if they did not? What properties of syllables make them useful for languages?

Note

1 The reader is reminded that signs are represented by English glosses in uppercase which may have lowercase pieces added (like "twist" and "x") to help identify different variants. See the discussion of annotation conventions in Chapter 1. Also, sign illustrations come from Signbank (www.aslsignbank.haskins.yale.edu) where readers can view movie clips to see the complete sign.

Further reading

Battison, R. (1978). *Lexical borrowing in American Sign Language*. Silver Spring, MD: Linstok Press.

Battison, R. (1980). Signs have parts. In C. Baker & R. Battison (Eds.), *Sign language and the deaf community* (pp. 35–51). Silver Spring, MD: National Association of the Deaf.

These works introduced the idea of constraints on the phonological formation of signs.

Brentari, D. (1998). *A prosodic model of sign language phonology*. Cambridge, MA: A Bradford Book.

This is an advanced analysis about the structure of signs in ASL that is currently very influential.

van der Hulst, H., & van der Kooij, E. (to appear). Phonological structure of signs – theoretical perspectives. In J. Q. Villanueva, R. Pfau, & A. Herrmann (Eds.), *The Routledge handbook of theoretical and experimental sign language research*. Abingdon, England: Routledge.

This is an overview chapter that summarizes much work on the phonological structure of signs.

Pfau, R., Steinbach, M., & Woll, B. (Eds.). (2012). *Sign language – an international handbook*. Berlin, Germany: Walter de Gruyter.

This large handbook has extensive information about the structure of different sign languages. Section A (Chapters 2–4) contains three chapters about different areas of phonology.

Sandler, W. (1986). The spreading hand autosegment of American Sign Language. *Sign Language Studies, 50*, 1–28.

Sandler, W. (2010). Prosody and syntax in sign languages. *Transactions of the Philological Society, 108*(3), 298–328.

This work presents an overview of prosody in sign languages, as discussed in Section 2.5.

Sandler, W. (2017). The challenge of sign language phonology. *Annual Review of Linguistics*, *3*, 43–63. doi:10.1146/annurev-linguistics-011516-034122
This article presents interesting similarities and differences between sign language phonology and spoken language phonology.

Stokoe, W. C., Casterline, D., & Croneberg, C. (1965). *A dictionary of American Sign Language on linguistic principles.* Washington, DC: Gallaudet College Press.
This is the first major work to treat a sign language in linguistic terms. It is a dictionary and also includes proposals about the phonological structure of ASL.

Bibliography

Corina, D. (1996). ASL syllables and prosodic constraints. *Lingua*, *98*, 73–102.

van der Hulst, H. (1993). Units in the analysis of signs. *Phonology*, *10*, 209–242.

Liddell, S. (1984). THINK and BELIEVE: sequentiality in American Sign Language. *Language*, *60*, 372–392.

Nespor, M., & Sandler, W. (1999). Prosody in Israeli Sign Language. *Language and Speech*, *42*, 143–176.

Chapter 3

Morphology

In this chapter, we continue our discussion of sign language grammar, turning to the domain of *morphology*. Morphology is the study of words, so in this chapter, we will look at how words are made in American Sign Language (ASL). We will discuss the ways that new words are formed, how words are modified, and the role of iconicity in ASL. The chapter also includes discussion of the way that the signing space is integrated in signs, and some morphological devices that seem to be special to sign languages.

3.1 What is morphology?

Morphology is the branch of linguistics that studies how words are formed from component parts. A morpheme is generally described as a consistent pairing of form (e.g., a sequence of sounds or a combination of handshape, location, and movement) and meaning, but there are morphemes that change their form in different contexts as well as those that don't seem to have a consistent meaning.

In spoken languages such as English, there are many words that are themselves a single morpheme, such as "cat," "elephant," "and," and "behind." Bear in mind that in English, a morpheme can have one, two, or more syllables – they are completely different notions. Words that contain two morphemes include "cats," "walking," and "rewrite." The plural marking -s on "cats," the progressive -ing on "walking," and the prefix re- in "rewrite" contribute an additional morpheme that either makes a word fit a particular context (the usual role of inflectional morphology), or changes the word into a new type with a new meaning (the usual role of derivational morphology). In addition to inflectional and derivational morphology, word formation is a component of morphology. Word formation encompasses the various ways that new words are added to a language. We will discuss sign language examples of each of these types of morphology in reverse order in the subsequent sections.

3.2 Word formation

New words constantly enter the vocabulary of a language, and other words may decline in usage. Words also change their meaning over time. All of these are natural processes of language, and not the "corruption" of a language by "kids these days" as often bemoaned. There are a number of processes that are used by languages when they need new words. Oftentimes, the existing words are used in a new way. Sometimes a word is used by itself with a new meaning, such as "mouse" to refer to a computer's pointing device. At other times, words combine into new, compound words. Compounds in English include "blackboard," "low-fat," and "motion sensor" (note that spelling might be with a space, hyphen, or no space – spelling is not a good indication of compound status). Words can also be borrowed from another language; when this happens, they are generally pronounced in such a way as to fit the language they are borrowed into, such as when the original language form includes sounds that the borrowing language doesn't have. An example is the word "champagne," borrowed from French, which is pronounced in English with different vowels from those used in French, and a different final n-sound.

Frequently, the association between a word and its meaning is completely arbitrary, such as the fact that "cat" refers to domesticated felines in English. When new words enter a language, they may also be arbitrary, but they are also frequently motivated in some way, either by a kind of iconicity or by rules of word formation. For example, many words that start with "gl" in English have a common sort of meaning – think of "gleam," "glisten," "glitter," and "glamour." These words all convey a sense of brightness or shininess, which seems to be associated with the beginning "gl."

This pattern is known as an example of sound symbolism, and it is a type of iconicity, which in this context means that there is a partially nonarbitrary relationship between form and meaning. Many scholars think that iconicity plays a large role in the words of sign languages: it is possible to detect a link between form and meaning in many signs. We turn next to exploring this relationship. Following our discussion of iconicity, we will see how compounding works in ASL in Section 3.2.2, and then we will turn to a method of borrowing words, fingerspelling.

3.2.1 Iconicity

Before sign language research began in earnest, many people assumed that signs were like drawing in the air, or pantomime, and so completely iconic. This was one rationale that was given for looking down on sign languages, since arbitrariness in the relation between form and meaning had been taken to be a fundamental characteristic of language, distinguishing it from other communicative systems. Thus, early researchers made a point of emphasizing the often arbitrary link between form and meaning in signs. For example, they noted that there are signs for abstract concepts (e.g., admire, believe, decide); how could these be iconic? They noted that nonsigners could not guess the meaning of a large proportion of signs presented in an experiment. And they showed that even if there is some degree of motivatedness in signs, there is still a great deal of conventionality. For example, the sign for TREE in different sign languages may bear some resemblance to a stereotypical tree, for instance, a trunk, the height of a tree, or a common shape of tree, but the signs can still be very different from each other, showing that language-particular aspects are more important than the connection to the visual image.

More recently, researchers have been interested in exploring the motivatedness and iconicity in signs of different sign languages. Since it is now linguistically established without question that sign languages are full natural languages, exploring nonarbitrariness is not seen as a threat any longer. With this new viewpoint, it is clear that iconicity is prevalent in sign languages.

Let's start by considering some signs for abstract concepts, illustrated in Figure 3.1. In some cases, an iconic basis for the sign

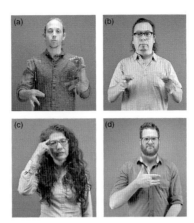

Figure 3.1 Signs for abstract concepts: (a) IF, (b) DECIDE, (c) THINK, and (d) FEEL. Images: ASL Signbank, 2018.

can be easily detected. For example, the sign used for "judge" (also used for "if," and glossed as IF in Signbank) employs an asymmetrical movement of two hands reminiscent of the movement of scales like the ones used to represent judgment; and DECIDE takes the "judge" sign and moves both hands sharply downward. Signs for mental concepts are generally made at the forehead (e.g., THINK, DREAMix), and signs for emotions are made at the heart (e.g., FEEL, AFFECTION). Although these concepts are abstract, there is a metaphor associated with each of them, and the signs are iconic to the metaphor.

There are many types of iconicity in the signs of ASL and other sign languages. Of course, this does not mean that nonsigners can easily guess what a sign means, but once they are told, the relationship between the sign and its meaning might be apparent (especially if they are familiar with the metaphors involved). Furthermore, the linguistic rules of each sign language still apply, and constrain the actual form used. Many iconic forms have a relationship to the classifier system, to be discussed in Section 3.5. How sign languages take advantage of the visual modality to productively employ iconicity linguistically is a matter of much current study.

3.2.2 Compounding

Like English, ASL permits productive compounding to produce
new words. Compounds can combine a noun with another noun
(e.g., BEDROOM), a verb with another verb (e.g., BRAINSTORM =
THINK and THROW), and other possible combinations (see
Figure 3.2). Particularly productive in ASL are compounds that
combine a lexical sign with a sign derived from the classifier system
(see Section 3.5) that depicts an aspect of the referent. For example,
CLOCK is composed of TIME plus what we might call DS_bl(round-
thing-on-vertical-surface), and COMPUTER-MOUSE is composed
of MOUSE plus DS_b3(manipulate-small-curved-object).

Compounds often are produced with a different rhythmical
pattern compared to words in a phrase. Well-known English examples are "(a) white hóuse" vs. "(the) White House," or "black
bóard" (a board that is black) vs. "bláck board" (a board for
writing on with chalk, no matter what color it is). However, different types of compounds work in different ways, so in English
"overdúe" is stressed on the second part, and "old-fáshioned"
is stressed on the first syllable of the second part. In ASL,

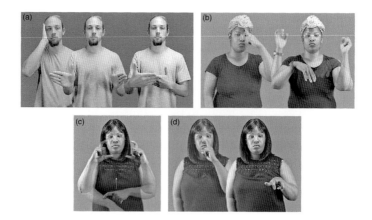

Figure 3.2 Signs produced by compounding: (a) BEDROOM, (b) BRAIN-
STORM (THINK THROW), (c) CLOCK (TIME DS_bl(round-
thing-on-vertical-surface)), and (d) COMPUTER-MOUSE (MOUSE
DS_b3(manipulate-small-curved-object)). Images: ASL Signbank,
2018.

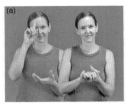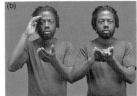

Figure 3.3 Compound with form reduction: (a) BELIEVEix and (b) BELIEVEb. Images: ASL Signbank, 2018.

compounds may be compressed in time and form, even losing so much as to form only one syllable in some cases. For example, the sign BELIEVE comes from a compound of THINK and MARRY. THINK is formed using movement of the ⚭ handshape toward the forehead, palm down. In the compound, the palm orientation turns to the contralateral side, and the movement toward the forehead becomes transitional; the primary movement of the sign is the movement of the hand from the forehead to the nondominant hand (in the part of the sign derived from MARRY). Sometimes, even the handshape of the first part changes to match the handshape of the second part (this is known as assimilation) – so the sign is made with only one handshape, ⚭. See the illustrations in Figure 3.3.

3.2.3 *Fingerspelling and initialization*

Fingerspelling is the use of different handshapes representing letters of the English alphabet to spell out words. It is a way to convert English words into a form that can be pronounced in ASL, just as the English pronunciation is used when a word is borrowed from another language, like "champagne." Fingerspelling is often used for the names of places and people, particularly if the signs for these names are not likely to be known, or if there are no common signs. Fingerspelling is also used to borrow other words into ASL, such as technical terms.

Sometimes fingerspelled words are modified to better fit the phonology of ASL, particularly if they are commonly used. These are often known as fingerspelled loan signs, acknowledging both their source in fingerspelling and their modified sign-like form. Some examples include #BACK, #BANK, #EARLY, and #JOB (many researchers use the symbol # to indicate a fingerspelled loan sign, but this notation is not used in ASL Signbank, which does not include fingerspelled words).

Another way that words from English can be borrowed into ASL is through initialization. This is a process using the fingerspelling handshape of the first letter of an English word, incorporated into an ASL sign. Often, there is a group of such signs that have the same location and movement, but different handshapes, such as commonly used signs for CLASS, FAMILY, SOCIETY, and ASSOCIATION.

3.3 Derivation

The previous section on word formation showed some ways in which new words can enter into a language. If we evaluate the patterns of words that are already in a language, we may find two types of processes by which words are related to each other. One type, inflectional morphology, adjusts words so that they fit better into the grammatical context in which they are used. This type of process, inflection, will be discussed in Section 3.4. The second type is derivational morphology, the subject of the current section. Derivational morphology changes words so that they take on a new grammatical category·(for example, converting the English verb "read" to a noun used in a phrase like "the poetry reading (was successful)"), or significantly alters their meaning (such as converting a English verb like "zip" to its opposite sense with the prefix "un-", giving "unzip"). In ASL, there is a group of nouns and verbs that are considered related by derivational morphology, which we turn to now.

3.3.1 Noun–verb pairs

There is a set of signs in ASL where the form used in a nominal context and the form used in a verbal context are closely related. Examples include AIRPLANE and AIRPLANE-FLY, illustrated in Figure 3.4.

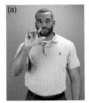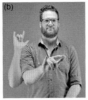

Figure 3.4 Noun/verb pair: (a) AIRPLANE and (b) AIRPLANE-FLY. Images: ASL Signbank, 2018.

It has been observed that there is a systematic difference between the noun and verb forms of these signs: the noun signs have a repeated, restrained movement, and the verb forms tend to have a single, unrestrained movement or a long, repeated movement. This is similar to the relationship between the English noun "prótest," which has stress on the first syllable, and the verb "protést," which has stress on the second syllable. Although the words are completely alike other than the stress pattern, we know that one is a verb and the other a noun. Similarly, the movement pattern allows signers to distinguish between the ASL noun AIRPLANE and the verb AIRPLANE-FLY.

The pattern that relates nouns and verbs is observed in a large number of cases of ASL, including those that have concrete objects such as AIRPLANE/AIRPLANE-FLY, CHAIR/SIT, and DRESS/WEAR. Note that the meaning of the verb is not always completely predictable from the meaning of the noun, although it is usually a prototypical action done with/by the noun; for example, the sign WEAR applies to various kinds of clothing, not only dresses. The ASL sign BOOK involves short repeated movement; a long movement in the opening direction is OPEN-BOOK and a long movement in the closing direction is CLOSE-BOOK, but the sign for READ is completely different, although the prototypical action to carry out with a book is reading.

In addition to relating concrete objects and actions done with/by them, the same pattern can be found in some pairs of signs for abstract nouns and related verbs, such as ACCEPT/ACCEPTANCE, DEVELOP/DEVELOPMENT, and JOIN/PARTICIPATION. Such signs are described in some of the linguistic literature, but some of them may be restricted to certain types of signing (also known as registers).

The noun–verb contrast as discussed here has been described in numerous papers and books about ASL. However, it should be noted that a visible contrast between items in nominal and verbal contexts is not always seen. For example, the sign EAT is produced with small repeated movements and it is not at all clear that there is a different sign for the noun "food." This could be an example of what is known as "zero derivation" or "conversion," where a word can be used in two word classes ("parts of speech") without any distinction. In English, this frequently happens in adjective/noun pairs, such as "green," which can be used as an adjective ("a green park") or a noun ("a town green").

Linguists have asked whether in ASL the noun is derived from the verb, or the verb is derived from the noun. In English, examples like "a reading" show that it is possible to derive a noun ("reading") from a verb ("read"); it is also possible to derive a verb, such as "shelve," from a noun ("shelf"). For ASL, however, it was proposed that neither the verb form nor the noun form is derived from the other. On the other hand, the variety of abstract nouns available do seem to be derived from the verbs, which may well be more common and well known.

3.3.2 Other types of derivation

A few other types of derivation have been studied, but not intensively. In spoken languages, derivation is frequently signaled by affixation, the addition of a morpheme to a root, such as the English prefix "un-" in words like "undo," or the suffix "-able" as in "likeable." In sign languages, affixation is observed only rarely; more frequently, derivation is signaled by a change in the movement of a sign or, in some cases, its handshape.

ASL uses affixation to negate some signs, such as DON'T-KNOW, DON'T-LIKE (illustrated in Figure 3.5a), and DON'T-WANT. The affix involves a movement away and a twisting wrist; if the root sign has a handshape change, the affix will reverse it (for example, LIKE, shown in Figure 3.5b, has a

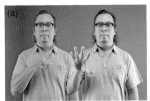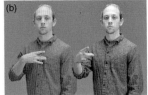

Figure 3.5 Negative affixation: (a) DON'T-LIKE and (b) LIKE. Images:
ASL Signbank, 2018.

closing handshape change, while the negative suffix applied to
this sign has an opening handshape change). There are additional phonological changes that may cause the negated sign
to have only one syllable, rather than one for the root plus one
for the affix (see Chapter 2, Section 2.6, for more on syllables in
ASL). While a similar pattern can be seen across several signs,
its productivity is very limited and this negative affix cannot be
added to most verbs.

It has also been proposed that ASL uses an affix for "-er" to
produce signs like TEACHER from TEACH. However, this form
is identical to the sign PERSONb, so it might be more appropriate
to analyze the combination as a compound rather than a process
of affixation.

Although affixation is clearly limited in ASL, changing the form
of a sign by altering its movement or handshape is a more common
means of derivation. We have already discussed the use of movement
differences to mark nouns and verbs. Another example involves
changing the movement of adjective signs to mark subtle meaning
differences, such as "deep-blue," "bright-red," or "very-slow."

It is also possible to change the handshape of a sign to derive
another form using a process known as numeral incorporation.
By this process, signs for DAY, WEEK, NEXT-DAY, DAY-AGO,
MONTH, MINUTE, and HOUR can indicate the number of
days, weeks, etc. Signers vary in the limits that are placed on
which numbers can be incorporated in each sign, but examples
like NINE-HOURS, THREE-DAYS, and EIGHT-MONTHS
(shown in Figure 3.6) are common.

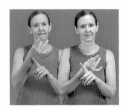

Figure 3.6 Numeral incorporation: EIGHT-MONTHS. Image: ASL Signbank, 2018.

3.4 Inflection

As mentioned earlier, inflection is a process that changes the form of a word so that it better fits the grammatical context. In English, the affix "-s" is added to verbs in the third-person singular context, such as "s/he runs" vs. "I/you/we/they run." Other languages, such as Spanish, change the form of articles (words for "the," "a"'), demonstratives (words for "this," "those"), and adjectives to agree in gender with the noun they appear with. This grammatical gender marking is a largely arbitrary division of nouns into "masculine" and "feminine," but the labels are extensions to nongendered items (like *el sol* "the sun" (masc.) vs. *la luna* "the moon" (fem.)) from the forms used with male and female humans.

Some languages make extensive use of inflection, with many different verb forms based on such characteristics as the participants, and the temporal features of the verb context, or multiple genders and/or case marking used with nouns. Other languages make little to no use of inflectional morphology, relying on other aspects of the grammar to make relevant distinctions. Sometimes people think that the complex inflectional systems of languages like Latin make those languages "more grammatical," and languages without such systems are somehow less complete. However, this is not an accurate notion. ASL (like other sign languages) has several types of inflectional morphology, although the way the system works in ASL is completely different from English.

3.4.1 Verbal morphology

Under the category of verbal morphology, we will discuss two kinds of inflection found on verbs in ASL: agreement and aspect. Agreement refers to the kind of process that makes a verb "agree" with its subject (and, in the case of ASL, its object). In English, it is agreement that gives us the third-person singular form "-s" on verbs. Aspect has to do with the temporal characteristics of the event described: is it an event that happened once, or multiple times? Is it a completed event or an ongoing one? In English, inflectional morphology is used to mark progressive aspect, as in "she is walking" (vs. "she walks" or "she walked"); English also marks verb tense distinguishing past ("-ed") from nonpast (no affix).

3.4.1.1 Agreement

In ASL, the verb agreement process makes use of locations in space that are also relevant for the pronominal system. We start by describing these spatial loci and how pronouns are signed, and then show how verb agreement works.

The sign meaning "I/me" (glossed IX_1) is produced by a signer pointing to their own chest, much like a common version of the pointing-to-self gesture that nonsigners produce. Pronouns or agreement forms that refer to the speaker/signer are called first person. A signer can point toward their addressee (the person they are talking to, also called second person) to produce a pronoun that means "you." What about third person, the equivalent of "she/he/it"? If a person is present in the discourse context, but not the addressee, the signer can point to that person's actual location. If the person is not present, another location will be used for the point. It could be a place the person often occupies (e.g., their desk if the signers are in a school or work environment), or it can be a completely arbitrary location. Generally, signers might use contrasting locations on the right and left side of their signing space to contrast different referents. In principle, any location could be used, but signers don't tend to distinguish more than two or three locations in space for different referents. Pointing signs are glossed as IX followed by the referent being pointed to within parentheses; e.g., IX(Lee). When a signer wants to refer to more than one person, usually an arc is added to the pointing sign (IXarc).

The locations in signing space that are used for pronouns are often referred to as *loci*. These loci are also used in the verb agreement system. When a verb is marked for agreement, it usually starts in the position of the locus associated with its subject and moves toward the position of the locus associated with its object. For example, the ASL sign ASKonex is illustrated in Figure 3.7. The photo shows the *citation form*, that is, the form that has no special modification to show agreement. It is also the form that would be used with a first-person subject and a second-person object: "I ask you." If the subject is second person and the object is first person, the whole sign would be turned around to face the signer, starting at a position away from the signer (in the direction of the addressee), and moving toward the signer (the first-person locus). Similarly, if the subject is first person and the object is a third person whose locus has been associated with a location on the signer's right side, the sign would move from a position close to the signer's body, toward the position on the right side. For this sign, both the orientation of the hand and the movement will change to indicate the subject and the object.

Not all verbs in ASL show agreement in the same way. There is a set that behaves more-or-less as just described, including HELPstr, SHOW, GIVE, LEND, and FEED, but even among these there are some differences (e.g., GIVE modifies its movement path, but not its orientation). The verbs that mark agreement with subject/object are *transitive* verbs, which have two or three arguments (a subject,

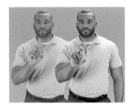

Figure 3.7 ASL sign that can participate in verb agreement: ASKonex. Image: ASL Signbank, 2018.

an object, and possibly an indirect object). Another set of verbs is called *backward* verbs because they start at the locus of their object and end at the locus of their subject. The signs INVITE, COPY (shown in Figure 3.8), and STEAL are among the backward verbs.

Agreement as just described involves verbs that (usually) have a human subject and object (indirect object in the case of ditransitive verbs). However, if a verb denotes a spatial relationship such as movement between a source location and a goal location, then these spatial loci will be the basis for agreement. For example, the sign GOix indicates movement from one place to another. It can be modified to indicate the beginning location at the beginning of the sign, and the ending location at the end of the sign, for example to convey, "She went from Boston to Los Angeles." Verbs whose movement through signing space represents movement through physical space are known as *spatial* verbs. In addition to representing movement through space, spatial verbs can indicate a location in space, such as the sign STAY, which can be modified to show the place where the referent is located by the location where it is signed (not the path movement between two locations). Loci can also be used to indicate the location of an event, such as when the sign LEAVE-ALONE is signed in the location of something to mean "leave this thing here alone."

Some verbs are not modified to indicate agreement with subject/object or with spatial locations. Verbs that are not modified are generally referred to as *plain* verbs. Some of the verbs that fail to take modification are described as body-anchored: that is, they involve an obligatory contact with the body. Verbs such as

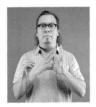

Figure 3.8 ASL sign that shows backward agreement: COPY. Image: ASL Signbank, 2018.

LIKE and LOVE are never modified for agreement. Intransitive verbs (verbs with only a subject, like LAUGH, SLEEP, RUN, or DANCE) do not agree with their subject, but sometimes they can be modified for a spatial location (e.g., ARRIVE).

The system of verb agreement described here has been extensively studied by sign linguists, but they do not all agree on the analysis. Some researchers do not think the system is actually like the processes of agreement found in spoken language. They might use the term *indicating verbs* rather than agreeing verbs to refer to this process. The term *directionality* is sometimes used as a neutral form to refer to the process without committing to one analysis or another. How the different verbs are divided up into those that are modified and those that are not is another topic of much discussion in the sign language linguistics literature. Very similar processes are found in almost all of the (established) sign languages of the world that have been studied to date, so another issue for discussion has been to consider what can explain this apparent sign language universal phenomenon.

3.4.1.2 Aspect

Verbs in ASL can be modified in another way aside from the process known as verb agreement: they can show certain aspects of the way that the event they describe unfolds over time. In many spoken languages, verbs are modified to indicate *tense* – whether the event described is in the present, past, or possibly in the future. In ASL, this kind of temporal marking is accomplished by separate words or phrases that set the scene in a sentence or a group of sentences. However, ASL also has a morphological process for indicating another kind of temporal relationship known as *aspect*.

There are two phenomena that fall under the category of aspect marking in ASL (and other sign languages). First, we will describe how individual signs might take a particular form according to whether they are (generally) used to describe ongoing events versus events that have a clear termination. Then, we will turn to what is probably a more common usage, when a sign is modified to show more about the temporal properties of a particular event being described in a particular utterance.

The term *telicity* is used to divide verbs into those that describe events that have a natural endpoint, such as "die," which are called *telic*; and those that denote events that are continuous, such as "walk," which are called *atelic*. More properly, a predicate or a phrase that includes a verb describes such events, since we can see that "walk in the park" has no natural, necessary endpoint but "walk to the park" is an activity that ends once the park is reached. In ASL, many verbs that describe telic events are produced with a clear endpoint in the sign, while those that describe atelic events are continuous (the signer stops eventually, but the sign could be produced with several cycles). For example, consider the signs ARRIVE and RUNasym, shown in Figure 3.9. ARRIVE is produced with a clear endpoint, which happens when the back of the dominant hand hits the open palm and fingers of the nondominant hand. On the other hand, RUNasym is produced with repeated handshape change which could happen two, three, or four times. These characteristics of the form of the signs correspond with their telicity: "arrive" is a telic predicate, which has a natural endpoint, but "run" (on its own) is atelic.

The notion that verbs indicate their telicity by their form is not without exception. There are verbs that do not follow the expected pattern; for example, SLEEP is atelic, but the sign is produced with a clear endpoint. However, the pattern can be seen across a number of signs and it also holds across different sign languages.

Going beyond the telicity of events, if a signer wishes to show that a particular activity was repeated, the sign can be modified through *reduplication* (repetition) or other changes of the movement. This is true even for signs whose base form includes an

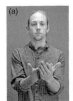

Figure 3.9 Telic and atelic signs: (a) ARRIVE and (b) RUNasym. Images: ASL Signbank, 2018.

endpoint. So, if the sign ARRIVE is repeated, it might be used to mean "arrive many times," "many people arrive," or "arrive in different places," depending on how it is signed. Even though the sign RUNasym is naturally repeated, it can be extended for a longer period to mean "run a long time," or "run every day," or "run over and over again." Different forms of reduplication are used to indicate different kinds of variations on a basic activity. In fact, it's even possible to use no movement at all on a sign to modify its meaning; the sign LOOK can be produced without movement to indicate a meaning like "stare." Many verbs that do not participate in the agreement process can be modified in the ways just described for aspect. This is a rather productive process in ASL.

3.4.2 Pluralization

The previous subsection discussed several kinds of inflectional modification that apply to verbs in ASL. What about nouns – are there any inflections on nouns? A candidate for such an inflection is pluralization, which is often said to be marked on ASL nouns by reduplication, or repetition of the noun. An example of this is the pair of signs CHILD and CHILDREN, illustrated in Figure 3.10. The sign CHILD is made with a single downward movement of one hand. The sign CHILDREN is made by moving the hand(s) downward, then arcing slightly up and to the ipsilateral side and down again twice (for a total of three movements downward), with one or both hands. CHILDREN is like a repeated version of CHILD, although the repetitions are not produced in the same spatial location but distributed.

Reduplication to mark pluralization is a common feature of many languages, so it would not be surprising to see that sign languages take advantage of this type of production. However, pairs like the one in Figure 3.10 are actually quite rare in ASL; most signs cannot be pluralized by adding reduplication. Instead, number information is usually carried by other signs, such as numerals (ONE, TWO, etc.) or quantifiers (ALL, MANY, SEVERAL).

Because the signs that can be reduplicated to make plurals are very limited, it is not clear whether it is appropriate to call such reduplication an inflectional process in ASL. In any case, you should understand that some signs come in such singular/plural pairs, but the process is not general.

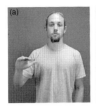 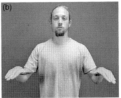

Figure 3.10 Potential plurality marking: (a) CHILD and (b) CHILDREN.
Images: ASL Signbank, 2018.

3.5 Classifiers

ASL (like other sign languages) has a highly productive process to form complex signs that represent events and states (generally considered to be predicates). The process involves the use of specific handshapes to represent particular classes of elements; for this reason, the handshapes have been analyzed as *classifiers*, and many researchers call the constructions *classifier constructions*. First, we will explain a bit more about what these signs look like, and then we will discuss the question of how they are analyzed linguistically.

In lexicalized signs, the handshape, movement, and location are phonological aspects that are not commonly analyzed as morphemic (that is, they are the sublexical components and do not carry their own regular independent meaning). However, in classifier constructions, each of these components is meaningful. In particular, the handshape is used to represent specific semantic classes. There are several different types of classifiers. Although different researchers use different groupings, we will adopt the following classification of classifiers:

a   *Whole entity*: The handshape represents an item from a semantic group; for example, the 🖐 handshape represents vehicles (cars, busses, boats), the 👆 handshape represents upright beings (people, bears), and the (bent-👆) handshape represents small animals (cats, birds). Movement of the classifier through signing space represents the movement of the entity represented by the handshape.
b   *Handling*: The handshape mimics a hand holding an item; for example, the (flat-✍) handshape represents holding flat items

with some thickness (such as a book, a hard drive, or a cereal box), and the (🖐) handshape represents holding items with a cylindrical handle (such as a hammer or a potato masher). When a classifier construction uses a handling classifier, it expresses the meaning that an agent manipulates an object in a particular way.

c   *Body-part*: The handshape represents a part of the body of a human or animal, and by inference, the whole being to which the body part belongs; for example, the (🖐) handshape represents the legs of a human, and the (spread-🖐) handshape represents the claws of an animal. The classifier construction using a body part classifier indicates the actions of the person or animal represented, with a focus on the movement of that part.

d   *Size-and-shape specifier*: Size-and-shape specifiers are used to describe an object rather than the movement of an object. The handshape represents size and/or shape; for example, the (🖐) handshape indicates a circular object, and both hands in the (🖐) handshape can represent a cylindrical object by moving apart from each other, outlining the size and shape of the cylinder (for example, a pipe, broom handle, or stroller handle).

Already it should be clear that classifier constructions are quite complex, but in fact there is more to the story. While the handshape represents an entity and the movement (except for size and shape specifiers) represents the movement of an entity, the manner of the sign movement represents the manner of movement being depicted.

Classifier constructions can involve one or two hands. When both hands are whole entity classifiers, the relationship between the hands represents the relationship between the entities referred to. For example, one hand might represent a person and the other a dog; or one hand might represent a tree and the other a bird perched on a branch of the tree. The two hands can each represent handling the same object (e.g., a lawn mower handle), or different objects (e.g., one hand holding a large hunk of cheese and the other holding a knife to cut off a piece); it's also possible for one hand to be a whole entity classifier while the other is a handling classifier (e.g., a board that an agent is using a saw to cut). In body-part classifiers, if two hands are used they might indicate two entities (e.g., two people represented by their legs), or two limbs of a single entity (e.g., two front legs of a bear). As already mentioned, in size-and-shape specifiers, two hands can be used to show the extent of an object through the movement of the hands; or, the two hands can represent two different objects (e.g., the placement of two buttons on a shirt).

When two hands are used in a classifier construction, generally the first sign that is produced is a *ground* and the second is a *figure*; the figure acts against the ground, such as walking on a surface or in front of something, placing an object on top of another one, or bumping an object against another.

Why might the term classifier be an appropriate label for such constructions? Spoken languages have several different types of constructions that are called classifiers, but the sign language structure is most similar to what are known as *verbal classifiers*, which are found in many Native American languages. These constructions involve a morpheme that represents a class of nouns being attached to a verbal stem, which is a very similar notion to the sign language classifiers. Linguists have considered the similarity and differences between sign language classifier constructions and verbal classifiers in spoken languages, and a detailed analysis is likely to be proposed in the future.

The information expressed by classifier constructions, especially their location, movement, and manner components, can be rich and difficult to break down into component parts. Furthermore, there is often more complexity expressed through the signer's nonmanual marking including facial expressions and body movement. For this reason, some researchers prefer to use the term *depiction* for these structures, which indicates that the way the signer expresses the meaning is meant to evoke a mental image in the receiver. Other researchers use the term "polycomponential" to emphasize the point that these constructions are highly complex and can be broken down into component parts. Such proposals sometimes involve rejecting the classifier label altogether, but other researchers are comfortable talking about such structures as a combination of classifiers and depiction. In some ways, these structures resemble the use of vocal intonation and body movement with spoken words in expressive quotations and narratives, and these are the contexts in which they are most frequently used in ASL as well.

The term depiction can also be applied to other structures found in ASL and other sign languages, known as Constructed Action and Constructed Dialogue. In these constructions, like classifiers, the signer's body, facial expression, and the manner of articulating signs are used to depict an intended meaning. Constructed Dialogue is used to report the speech, signing, or thoughts of a referent, and Constructed Action reports actions through showing them rather than telling about them. As with classifier constructions, multiple accounts have been proposed for these kinds of structures, so we must wait for a complete theory in the future. Meanwhile, we would like to point out that skilled use of classifier constructions, constructed action, and constructed dialogue are important parts of ASL poetry, storytelling, and other literary genres.

3.6 Conclusion

ASL, like other sign languages, has an interesting combination of characteristics. Many signs are formed of a single morpheme (which is also expressed in a single syllable), and there are few affixation processes. However, because of the ways that verbs and classifier predicates can be inflected, there are some signs that have multiple morphemes. The types of grammatical morphology in ASL are rather different from those found in English: English has productive noun pluralization, and verbs mark tense and agreement, while ASL marks person on verbs but also locative agreement and aspect but not tense. Some people have mistakenly characterized sign languages as lacking grammar because of these differences, but the reality is simply a different set of grammatical rules. In the next chapter, we will turn to looking at how the grammatical rules apply in the formation of sentences.

Discussion questions

1   Does ASL have parts of speech (or grammatical categories)? How can you tell?
2   How is verb agreement in ASL similar to and different from agreement in spoken languages?
3   What ways are classifiers like those found in spoken languages? How are they like depiction?
4   What does the study of sign language morphology tell us about language structure?
5   Suppose you discovered a sign language in which all words have only one morpheme. What would you conclude about this language?

Further reading

Aronoff, M., Meir, I., & Sandler, W. (2005). The paradox of sign language morphology. *Language*, *81*(2), 301–344.
This article discusses advanced linguistic concepts about sign language morphology, and how it is similar to and different from the kinds of morphology seen in spoken languages.

Emmorey, K. (Ed.). (2003). *Perspectives on classifier constructions in sign languages*. Mahwah, NJ: Lawrence Erlbaum Associates.
This book contains a number of articles discussing the pros and cons of using the "classifier" label and analysis.

Lillo-Martin, D., & Meier, R. P. (2011). On the linguistic status of "agreement" in sign languages. *Theoretical Linguistics*, *37*, 95–141.
This article provides an overview of the analyses of verb agreement in sign languages.

Pfau, R., Steinbach, M., & Woll, B. (Eds.). (2012). *Sign language – An international handbook*. Berlin, Germany: Walter de Gruyter.
This large handbook has extensive information about the structure of different sign languages. Section B (Chapters 5–11) contains seven chapters about different areas of morphology.

Supalla, T., & Newport, E. L. (1978). How many seats in a chair? The derivation of nouns and verbs in American Sign Language. In P. Siple (Ed.), *Understanding language through sign language research* (pp. 91–132). New York, NY: Academic Press.
This chapter was the first to describe the regular formational relationship between nouns and verbs in ASL.

Bibliography

Abner, N. (2017). What you see is what you get.get: surface transparency and ambiguity of nominalizing reduplication in American Sign Language. *Syntax*, *20*(4), 317–352.

Aronoff, M., Meir, I., & Sandler, W. (2005). The paradox of sign language morphology. *Language*, *81*(2), 301–344.

Bellugi, U., & Newkirk, D. (n.d.). Formal devices for creating new signs in ASL. *Sign Language Studies*, *10*, 1–35.

Brentari, D., & Padden, C. (2001). Native and foreign vocabulary in American Sign Language: a lexicon with multiple origins. In D. Brentari (Ed.), *Foreign vocabulary in sign languages: a cross-linguistic investigation of word formation* (pp. 87–119). Mahwah, NJ: Lawrence Erlbaum Associates.

Fischer, S., & Gough, B. (1978). Verbs in American Sign Language. *Sign Language Studies*, *7*, 17–48.

Friedman, L. (1975). Space, time, and person reference in American Sign Language. *Language*, *51*, 940–961.

Meir, I. (2002). A cross-modality perspective on verb agreement. *Natural Language and Linguistic Theory*, *20*(2), 413–450.

Padden, C. A. (1983). *Interaction of morphology and syntax in American Sign Language* (Ph.D. Dissertation). University of California, San Diego, CA.

Rathmann, C., & Mathur, G. (2002). Is verb agreement the same cross-modally? In R. P. Meier, K. Cormier, & D. Quinto-Pozos (Eds.), *Modality and structure in signed and spoken languages* (pp. 370–404). Cambridge, MA: Cambridge University Press.

Chapter 4

Syntax

4.1 Introduction: what is syntax?

As mentioned in Chapter 2, grammar includes all of the components of a given language – phonology, morphology, syntax, and semantics. We commonly understand "grammar" as prescriptive grammar, i.e., what is prescribed about how one should or should not construct a given sentence in our language. For example, one prescriptive rule in American English is that a sentence cannot end with a preposition, as in "What will you cut the paper with?" or "I would like to know where the beef came from." However, such sentences are quite natural in spoken English. Another prescriptive rule of grammar in American English concerns the use of double negation, the use of which is assumed to then create a positive interpretation as in "I don't *not* like him." However, in nonstandard dialects of English and many languages, sentences like "Nobody didn't eat the pie" retain their negative interpretation rather than becoming positive in interpretation. In standard English, many people would prescriptively judge the double negation to be ungrammatical or "bad English" if the negative interpretation is retained.

Linguists are not concerned about these prescriptive rules, but instead look at how native speakers of a language use their language every day. The linguistic approach is to describe the implicit rules that govern linguistic constructs, which are called *descriptive rules.* In other words, we are interested in describing what occurs in a given language, not passing judgment. For example, in English, we know that adjectives precede the noun that they modify, as in "I saw the <u>red</u> box." In other languages such as French and Basque, the adjectives typically follow the noun. Another rule in English would be that wh-words such as "who," "what," and "why" generally occur at the beginning of the question as in "<u>Who</u> does John want to meet?" or "<u>What</u> did John buy at the store?" (such questions are known as *wh-questions*). Since we understand "who" and "what" as referring to the object of "meet" and "buy," respectively, linguists have proposed that these words move from their base position (where a nonquestion word would appear) to the front of the sentence. On the other hand, in Japanese, the equivalent words remain in their base position, which we call *in situ*. Such a question would look like this in English: "John bought <u>what</u> at the store?" We can only use this kind of structure in English under very particular kinds of situations (such as surprise or requesting clarification), but it is the normal way to ask a question in Japanese. As we will see later in this chapter, ASL allows both structures for regular wh-questions. These examples should help you realize that when we talk about grammatical rules in this chapter (and throughout the book), we have in mind these kinds of rules that native speakers know implicitly.

4.1.1 Overview of the chapter

Syntax is the study of the descriptive rules that are needed to build a sentence in a given language. In Chapter 2, we looked at the rules for producing a syllable, and in Chapter 3, we looked at the rules for building a word in ASL. Now, we will look at some basic components of ASL syntax and learn how to build a sentence.

In the following section, word order in ASL will be discussed, with an eye toward understanding that ASL allows a degree of flexibility in word ordering, but this flexibility is related to particular aspects of the way a sentence fits with the context, known as discourse information. Section 4.3 illustrates the importance of nonmanuals (designated "facial expressions") in ASL syntax by looking at several different structures that use the nonmanual marker brow raise. In this section we will look at how word order and nonmanuals combine to create yes/no questions, conditionals, and topic structures in ASL. Then, in Section 4.4, interrogative questions in ASL are discussed. Finally, the last section deals with negation, where we discuss an interesting observation about how the interpretation of a sentence changes depending on the position of a negative sign.

4.2 Word order in ASL

All languages are based on a simple, basic word order with respect to the grammatical subject (S), object (O), and verb (V). There are six possible combinations of these three elements: SOV, SVO, VSO, VOS, OVS, and OSV. How do we know which word order a given language follows, especially if the language uses more than one word order in certain contexts? We look at a simple, neutral sentence such as "I like apples," with no added intonation, discourse, or syntactic factors that may affect the ordering of the sentence. In English, the ordering for "I like apples" is SVO. In Japanese, it would be SOV, which using English words to represent Japanese would appear as "I apples like." English is known as a strict SVO language, because most of the time this order is used. However, once we look beyond the basic neutral sentences, there are some contexts in which the object occurs in a different position, namely sentence-initial. For example, "Chocolate, I like!" is grammatical in certain discourse contexts. ASL has the same basic word order as in English, SVO, but this is not because ASL is derived from or a signed form of English. ASL also permits variation in word order depending on the discourse context.

Although the basic word order can be determined for each language, sentences can also be used with a word order that does not follow the basic order. Oftentimes, these alternative orders are used in order to give some element in the sentence more prominence, or to highlight it and make it stand out. Another kind of variation might be used to put some part of the sentence in the background, or to remind the listener of something that has already been mentioned. These kinds of variations are ways that *information structure* affects sentential word order. The sentence from English given above, "Chocolate, I like!" is an example of this. By putting the object, "chocolate" at the beginning of the sentence, it receives a particular kind of emphasis. Notice that such a sentence would generally not be uttered out of the blue, but in a context where alternatives are being discussed. Perhaps it would be said in a contrasting setup, followed by, "but kale, I can't stand!" On the other hand, in English, it would also be possible to simply put stress on the word "chocolate" when it is in its usual, base position following the verb: "I like <u>chocolate</u>!"

Taking these kinds of factors into account, languages can be divided into two types: [+ plastic] and [- plastic]. Some languages use a specific position in a sentence for informational focus, i.e., intonational prominence or stress. Other languages allow different parts of the sentence to receive informational focus. "Plastic" refers to whether the language allows prominence to be realized in different positions (this is [+plastic]) or not (this is [- plastic]). If a language must keep stress in a particular position, then it will allow different word orderings so that the word or phrase that should be stressed appears in the correct position. If a language allows stress to vary, then there is not much need for changing the word order.

ASL is a [- plastic] language, as Russian and Catalan also are. Such languages must shift the ordering of syntactic elements in a sentence in order to ensure that the phrase receiving the informational focus is in clause-final position. English is a [+ plastic] language, along with Dutch and German, so the intonational pitch cooccurs with the phrase being prominently focused, wherever it is. Let's see how this works in ASL and English. In (1) below, we see the English sentence, "The dog chewed up my shoes." If one wants to bring into informational focus a particular word, it would be intonationally stressed with a pitch, as seen below by the use of underlined words.

1   a   The <u>dog</u> chewed up my shoes
     b   The dog <u>chewed up</u> my shoes
     c   The dog chewed up <u>my</u> shoes
     d   The dog chewed up my <u>shoes</u>

For ASL, the word order has to be shifted around to allow the word receiving informational focus to occur in clause-final position, so we would see analogous sentences to the ones above as shown in (2) below.[1]

2   (compare to (1a)):

$$\underline{\hspace{5cm}}\overset{\text{br}}{}$$

a   CHEW-UP POSS_1 SHOES IX <u>DOG</u>   or

$$\underline{\hspace{5cm}}\overset{\text{br}}{}$$

POSS_1 SHOES CHEW-UP, IX <u>DOG</u>

(compare to (1b)):

$$\underline{\hspace{2cm}}\overset{\text{br}}{} \underline{\hspace{3cm}}\overset{\text{br}}{}$$

b   IX DOG POSS_1 SHOES <u>CHEW-UP</u>   or

$$\underline{\hspace{4cm}}\overset{\text{br}}{}$$

POSS_1 SHOES, IX DOG <u>CHEW-UP</u>

(compare to (1c)):

$$\underline{\hspace{2cm}}\overset{\text{br}}{}$$

c   SHOES IX DOG CHEW-UP <u>POSS_1</u>

(compare to (1d)):

$$\underline{\hspace{2cm}}\overset{\text{br}}{}$$

d   IX DOG CHEW-UP POSS_1 <u>SHOES</u>

Now, notice the word orders for each of the sentences in (2), which, respectively, are VOS, OVS, SOV, OSV, OSV, and SVO. Five out of the six possible word orders are allowed in ASL; VSO is not allowed as it is considered ungrammatical in any possible construction. Moreover, as mentioned earlier, the basic word order for ASL is SVO, but because it is a [– plastic] language, it allows other word orders to occur, depending on information structure. Notice the notation of "br" above certain words in the sentences. This stands for "brow raise," which is the nonmanual marking most typically associated with topicalization in ASL. The following two sections will touch upon this feature of ASL grammar.

4.3 Syntactic structures with brow raise

In most signed languages, the grammar includes *nonmanuals*, which are certain facial expressions that co-occur with a corresponding grammatical construction. These facial expressions are not affective in nature, but function as a required marker indicating what kind of syntactic construction is being expressed. Such nonmanuals include *brow raises (br)*, *brow furrows (bf)*, *head nods (hn)*, and *headshakes (hs)*; each one is associated with particular syntactic constructions such as polar questions (questions where the expected answer is "yes" or "no," also known as yes/no questions), wh-questions (questions that begin with what are known as "wh-words" due to the spelling of their English versions), copulas (sentences that equate two parts, such as "she is a doctor"), and negation (sentences with negative elements such as "no" and "never"), along with different movements of the nose and mouth that are more typically associated with semantic information.

Nonmanuals are an important part of distinguishing different syntactic structures which superficially may look the same. Some nonmanuals such as the brow raise are associated with more than one syntactic construction. Others, such as the brow furrow or headshake, are more typically associated with one type of syntactic constructions, i.e., wh-questions and negation respectively, which we will discuss later in this chapter. In this section we will review several types of structures that are used with brow raises.

4.3.1 Yes/no interrogatives

As shown below in (3), it is possible for two ASL sentences to have exactly the same lexical items and word order, being distinguished only by the "br" in (3b), which indicates that this is a yes/no question.

3   a   IX WILL BUY SHOES TODAY
      "She will buy shoes today."

                                 br
      b   IX WILL BUY SHOES TODAY
        "Will she buy shoes today?"

In English, an auxiliary verb such as "did," "do," and "will" is required when creating a yes/no question as in "Did you buy the cheese?" or "Will she buy shoes today?" English also allows for the formation of yes/no questions using intonation alone, as in "You going to class today?" However, ASL uses nonmanuals to let the addressee know precisely what type of sentence is being expressed, in this case, a yes/no question rather than a statement.

4.3.2 Conditionals

Another type of ASL sentence that uses brow raise is conditionals, a construction that indicates the possibility of an event occurring and a consequence of that event. As we see in the two sentences below in (4), although they have the exact same manual signs, one is distinguished only by the "brow raise," which indicates that this is a conditional structure and therefore has a different interpretation.

4   a   RAIN TOMORROW, GAME CANCEL
          "It will rain tomorrow so the game is canceled."

          _____br
     b   RAIN TOMORROW, GAME CANCEL
          "If it rains tomorrow, the game will be canceled."

There are other complex constructions such as rhetorical questions (which the speaker answers themselves), wh-clefts (a way to highlight certain information in a sentence), or time adverbials (phrases that indicate the time of an event) that also utilize the brow raise nonmanual, but they will not be discussed in this chapter. The interested reader is encouraged to read more on this topic, which reveals a complex interaction of word order, nonmanuals, and semantic interpretation. The following sections will illustrate examples of such complexity using structures involving topicalization, wh-questions, and negation.

4.3.3 Topicalization

In the previous subsections, we talked about the use of raised eyebrows to indicate a yes/no question or a conditional construction.

Another syntactic construction that requires the use of "br" is *topicalization*, in which a particular part of the sentence is marked as a topic. Any part of the sentence in ASL can be topicalized – the subject, the object, verb phrase, or an adjunct phrase (adverb phrase, adjective phrase, location phrase). Topicalization includes the movement of a syntactic element to the front (or beginning) of a sentence and highlighting it as "old or previously discussed" information. For instance, consider the conversation in (5) below, a conversation about cheese. In the last line we can see that "goat cheese" has undergone topicalization: it appears at the beginning of the sentence and is marked with "br" as the topic. This topicalization is allowed because "goat cheese" is not new information but was previously mentioned in the discourse. If Speaker A had topicalized "goat cheese" in the first line, moving it to the front of the sentence, this would be considered ungrammatical since this is new information which cannot be topicalized. New information or pragmatically neutral information is typically presented in SVO order.

5   Discussion of cheese between A and B:
Speaker A: IX_1 REALLY LIKE CHEESE.
        "I really like cheese."

Speaker B: OH-YES, IX_1 LOVE CHEESE.
        "Oh yes, I love cheese."

        IX_1 EAT CHEESE DAILY.
        "I eat cheese every day."
        _____ bf
        TYPE IX LIKE?
        "What kind do you like?"

Speaker A: IX_1 LIKE ALL, ONE IX_1 NOT FOND, GOAT
        I   like   all,   one   I   not   favorite goat
        CHEESE, BLEH
        cheese   yuck
        "I like them all, except one (kind), and that's goat cheese. Yuck!"
        _____ br

Speaker B: GOAT CHEESE, IX_1 KISS-FIST!
        "Goat cheese, I love (it)!"

Another example of topicalization is shown below in (6), this time with the verb phrase being fronted from its base position to produce VOS order.

6   (with previous discourse discussing someone's father building a house)

               br

BUILD HOUSE, POSS FAVORITE MAJOR JOB

"As for building houses, that's his preferred line of work."

ASL also allows two topics to occur in the same sentence as we can see in (7):

7   (talking about vegetables)

        br   br

VEGGIE,   CORNix, IX_1 EAT DAILY

"As for vegetables, corn, I eat this every day."

ASL has three types of topics which have been called "tm1," "tm2," and "tm3," illustrated in Figure 4.1; each has its own constellation of nonmanuals that co-occurs with a particular syntactic frame and identifies a set of relationships in the discourse. All of the previous examples use "tm1," which typically identifies an element moved from its base position. In the following sentence, the topicalized item has not been moved from its base position and instead is considered a topic that is *base-generated*, i.e., it appears in the front of the sentence and has a pronominal or clause-internal object that is related to the topic.

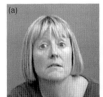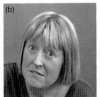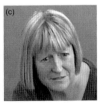

Figure 4.1 ASL nonmanual markers: (a) tm1, (b) tm2, and (c) tm3. Images: Copyright Wendy Sandler & Diane Lillo-Martin.

Such topics are marked by "tm2" (or "tm3"). They introduce new information about the discourse topic. The nonmanuals for "tm1" and "tm2" are almost the same, with just a subtle difference in the widening of the eyes and degree of head tilt, along with the requisite brow raises.

      <u>   tm2</u>

8   FRUIT, JOHN PREFER STRAWBERRY
     "As for fruit, John prefers strawberries."

The third topic marker, tm3, introduces a major shift in the discourse with referents that are known to both the speaker and addressee. The nonmanuals for this topic marker are quite distinct: raised brows, rapid head nods, and upper lip slightly raised. With this topic marker, the speaker identifies someone or something that they both know and then provides new information about this, as we see in (9).

      <u>   tm3</u>

9   BOB,   IX TOGETHER JOHN NOW
     (You know) Bob,   He together   John   now
     "(You know) Bob, he is dating John now."

Now, we have seen several examples of how a nonmanual works in tandem with word ordering to construct a particular type of syntactic structure in ASL, i.e., topics of different types. We next move on to another syntactic construction in which nonmanuals are used in an interrogative context, but in this case the use of the nonmanuals is more dependent on the grammatical structure than on discourse factors.

4.4 Wh-questions

We previously touched upon yes/no questions in an earlier section when discussing the importance of nonmanuals in ASL syntax. Yes/no questions are always marked by a brow raise that spans the full sentence, which is different from topics, where the brow raise only marks the topicalized item. Now, we will see another type of nonmanual, "brow furrow" depicted in Figure 4.2, which

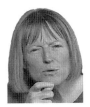

Figure 4.2 ASL brow furrow nonmanual marker. Image: Copyright Wendy Sandler & Diane Lillo-Martin.

marks wh-questions in ASL. The brow furrow nonmanual behaves quite differently from brow raises with either yes/no questions or topics.

Wh-questions are interrogative constructions in which a wh-word is used to create a question. Examples of wh-words in English are: "what," "who," "where," "when," "how," "which," and "why." All languages have wh-questions, but not necessarily the same number or form as in English. There has to be a syntactic mechanism for asking wh-questions in order to elicit information that one needs. However, some languages have one or two wh-words, which suffice for what they need to know, using the context in the discourse for identifying what kind of wh-question they are asking. A list of wh-words in ASL is provided in Table 4.1.

ASL has four wh-words for "what," each of which has its own role in the grammar. In the following subsections, we will discuss these wh-words and how wh-questions are created using them in ASL. After this section, the sentential structure for wh-questions will be explored, looking at the different positions in the syntax that wh-words can appear in, along with a discussion of multiple wh-questions in ASL.

Table 4.1   Wh-words in ASL

WHAT	WHAT-DO	WHAT-FOR
WHAT-PU	WHAT-FS	WHEN
WHERE	WHICH	WHO (several variants)
WHY	HOW	HOW-MANY

4.4.1 Marking the wh-question

There is some considerable debate in ASL linguistics research regarding the precise syntactic analysis for wh-question nonmanuals, of which there is a picture in the previous section. Some argue that there is a distinct nonmanual marker used for wh-topics that is separate from the one used for conventional wh-questions. We will not discuss this issue as it is beyond the scope of this chapter, but instead will focus on a traditional view of the wh-question nonmanual marking. ASL allows the nonmanual to suffice as the wh-morpheme, i.e. without an overt wh-word, as in (10), but in most contexts signers strongly prefer an overt wh-word to accompany the requisite "brow furrow" (11a, b). Signing a wh-question without the wh-question nonmanual marking, as in (11c), is possible, but it is considerably better when signed with the marking as in (11b).

<pre>
                    bf
10   a   TIME
         "What time is it?"

                          bf
     b   TYPE YOU WANT
         "What kind do you want?"

                          bf
11   a   YOUR NAME WHAT?
         "What is your name?"

                            bf
     b   WHERE YOUR HOME?
         "Where is your house?"

     c   ? WHERE YOUR HOME?
         "Where is your house?"
</pre>

As noted here and in other sections of this chapter, nonmanuals are an integral aspect of ASL syntactic structure, but we also need to look at the structures of the sentences themselves. In the following section we look at multiple distinct *WHAT* signs in ASL to better understand how these signs align themselves with particular grammatical constructions and interpretations.

4.4.2 The four WHATs

In ASL, there are four wh-signs for WHAT, all with the same basic underlying lexical interpretation. Each is signed in a different way and used with particular grammatical constructions. However, there are some subtle semantic distinctions that come with these grammatical constructions. They are signed as seen in Figure 4.3.

Not all of these signs are interchangeable. The first sign, WHAT-PU, is interchangeable with all the others and can be used in any possible wh-context as shown in (12). A direct wh-question is one that expects a content answer from the addressee. An indirect question uses question structure inside a larger sentence and does not necessarily expect a response. An echo question expresses surprise or a request for clarification. Finally, a D-linked question is one where the question is linked to some specific aspect of the previous discourse.

12 a   Simple, direct wh-question

⎯⎯⎯⎯⎯⎯⎯⎯⎯⎯⎯⎯⎯⎯bf

YOUR NAME WHAT-PU?
"What is your name?"

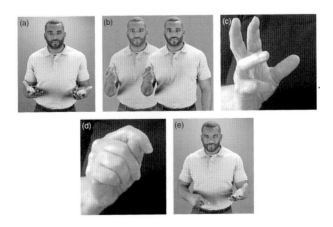

Figure 4.3 Four signs for "what" in ASL: (a) WHAT-PU, (b) WHAT-DO, (c) WHAT-FS, and (d) WHAT. Images (a), (b), (d): ASL Signbank, 2018; Image (c): Copyright Sandra Wood.

b   Indirect wh-question
IX_1 DON'T-KNOW WHAT-PU IX EAT
"I don't know what he ate/eats."

c   Echo/exclamation wh-question

<u>   bf</u>
JOHN BUY WHAT-PU?
"John bought what?!"

d   D-linked wh-question
With context of several books in front of person:

<u>   bf</u>
JOHN BUY WHAT-PU?
"What (book) did John buy?"

The next sign, WHAT-DO, is also capable of occurring in two of the sentence types listed above, direct questions and D-linked questions. It is not acceptable in indirect wh-questions (13a) and echo/exclamations (13b). We indicate that a sentence is not considered acceptable to native speakers/signers by putting the "*" in front of it. Notice that both indirect wh-questions and echo wh-questions do not contain the element of a direct query, so it can be concluded that WHAT-DO can only be used in the context of a question expecting a response.

13 a   *IX_1 DON'T-KNOW WHAT-DO IX EAT
"I don't know what he ate/eats."

<u>   bf</u>
b   *JOHN BUY WHAT-DO?!
"John bought what?!"

The third sign, WHAT-FS, is a fingerspelled loan sign, in which the fingerspelling of each letter has been phonologically merged together in a condensed version of the word, which now behaves as a sign (see Chapter 3 for discussion of fingerspelled loan signs). This sign is the opposite of WHAT-DO. It can only occur in indirect wh-questions and echo/exclamations.

    The last sign mentioned here will be WHAT. This is an old sign that is not in much use anymore, but it still has an interesting twist in its role with wh-questions in ASL. It is primarily used as a rhetorical question as in (14), which is not a direct question, but has an implied shared knowledge of the answer with the force of an assertion, rather than as an interrogative.

14 IX POSS WIFE, BIG HOUSE, FANCY CAR!
   She has a wife, a big house, and a fancy car!

   <u>   bf   </u>
   WHAT IX WANT?
   "What (more) does she want?"

However, WHAT can also occur in indirect questions (15a) and D-linked contexts (15b). When a wh-question is provided in a D-linked context, it relates back to previously mentioned information in the discourse. Thus, the range of the reference for D-linked phrases is limited to what is discourse-given, i.e., something that both the speaker and addressee already know. The question cannot be posed to someone out of the blue, for instance.

15 a IX_1 DON'T-KNOW WHAT IX EAT
     "I don't know what he ate/eats."

   b With context of several books in front of person:
     <u>   bf   </u>
     JOHN BUY WHAT?
     "What (book) did John buy?"

So far, we have discussed different contexts in which the four signs for WHAT can and cannot occur. This shows a complex interaction between the semantic structure and syntax in ASL grammar. Next, we will look at which position the wh-phrase can occur in for ASL and see how ASL fits within the universal paradigm.

4.4.3 Position of the wh-word

Looking across the world's languages, there are three primary positions within an interrogative sentence in which the wh-phrase is allowed to appear: *sentence-initially*, *in-situ*, and *sentence-finally*.

Typically, most languages choose one strategy for the positioning of the wh-phrase. In English, the wh-phrase is usually fronted, in the sentence-initial position, as in the sentence, "<u>What</u> did John eat yesterday?" However, it is also possible to produce a wh-question with the wh-word *in situ*, within the sentence, such as, "You ate <u>what</u> yesterday?" Such sentences are used in English to express surprise, request further information, or for other particular purposes.

However, other languages have different patterns. For instance, in Japanese, the wh-phrase remains in its base position, *in-situ*, even for ordinary questions. The object wh-phrase does not move to the front of the sentence. Furthermore, some languages allow more than one strategy; for example, French uses both the sentence-initial and *in-situ* strategies. ASL also allows multiple strategies.

In ASL, the *wh*-phrase can be in the *in-situ* position, as in (16a), or it can move to the front of the sentence, as in (16b). What is a bit unusual is that the wh-phrase can also occur in the sentence-final position, as in (16c). In many of the signed languages that have been studied, the wh-phrase often occurs sentence-finally. The sentence-final option is not usually seen in spoken languages.

16 a <u>   bf</u>
      JOHN SEE WHO YESTERDAY?
      "Who did John see yesterday?"

   b <u>   bf</u>
      WHO JOHN SEE YESTERDAY?

   c <u>   bf</u>
      JOHN SEE YESTERDAY WHO?

As we can see, there are a variety of strategies that ASL employs in the positioning of the wh-phrase. It is not clear why ASL prefers to utilize three strategies, instead of one or two. One more cross-linguistic strategy remains to be considered, regarding multiple wh-questions, which are interrogatives that have two or more wh-words. We will now move on to look at how ASL handles these.

4.4.4 Wh-doubling and multiple wh-questions

Up to this point, we have been discussing single wh-questions, but ASL also allows questions with more than one wh-phrase. There are two kinds of sentences that have more than one wh-phrase, and they are very different. One is *wh-doubling* and the other is *multiple wh-questions*.

In many sign languages (but not all), wh-doubling is a commonly used strategy. In doubling, a wh-phrase appears at the front of the sentence, and a copy of that wh-phrase appears at the end. In ASL, wh-doubling is a way to focus the wh-phrase for emphasis. Examples of wh-doubling are given in (17). In those examples of wh-doubling, the wh-phrases are always the same (WHO, WHO or WHAT, WHAT).

```
                               bf
17  a   WHO JOHN MARRY WHO?
        "Who did John marry??"
```

```
                                           bf
    b   WHAT-PU JOHN BUY YESTERDAY WHAT-PU?
        "What did John buy yesterday??"
```

In multiple wh-questions, the wh-phrases are not the same. These questions are about pairs of things, as in the English example, "Who is taking which class?" ASL allows multiple wh-questions in which there is one wh-phrase in sentence-initial position and another in sentence-final position, as illustrated in (18). These examples involve the first wh-phrase appearing at the front of the sentence, and the second wh-phrase at the end of the sentence.

```
                             bf
18  a   WHO BUY YESTERDAY WHAT-PU?
        "Who bought what yesterday?"
```

```
                        bf
    b   WHO JOHN GIVE WHAT-PU
        "What did John give to whom?"
```

We will see in the next section on negation that doubling is not unusual and it is a common strategy in ASL (and other sign languages) to provide emphasis or to focus information. A parallel between strategies for wh-questions and negation is commonly attested cross-linguistically and ASL fits within that paradigm.

4.5 Negation

All languages must have a way to express negation. For every utterance or proposition that is expressed in a positive sense, there is a mechanism for negating that positive proposition. For instance, "I have three apples" is a positive proposition. To negate this in English, we add a negative element such as "not" or "no" (among others), as in "I do not have three apples" or "I have no apples." There are different ways to express negation, but in all cases, the negative particle has *scope* over something in the sentence, indicating semantically that particular lexical item or proposition is being negated.

In this chapter, we will discuss four different negative lexical items in ASL: NOT, NEVER, NONEaltvar, and NOTHING-AT-ALL. The first two are sentential negators, which means that they make a whole sentence negative. The latter two are negators that modify the subject and/or object. Before we study the structure of these four negative lexical items, let's take a look at one defining hallmark of negation seen not only in ASL, but in all signed languages: negative nonmanuals.

4.5.1 Nonmanuals for negation

Negative signs are typically accompanied by a nonmanual negative marker. The nonmanual for negation in ASL is a headshake from side to side; it can stand alone or appear with a negative lexical item, as shown in (19). The negative nonmanual and negative lexical items serve to indicate the scope of negation, i.e., what part of the event in the utterance is being negated. In (19), the negative markers are used to negate the full sentence.

                                               <u>   neg</u>

19   a   IX_1 UNDERSTAND STORY
          "I did not understand the story."

                                                          neg
    b   IX_1 NOT UNDERSTAND STORY
        "I did not understand the story."

Most (but not all) signed languages employ the side-to side-headshake for negation but vary with respect to the additional use of other nonmanuals such as puffed cheeks or a backward head tilt at the same time. ASL typically indicates negation with a side-to-side headshake and furrowed brow; at times, two additional nonmanuals employing the mouth are included with the headshake: HS_{zig} (mouth is set in a bite and eyes are squinted) and HS_{swish} (mouth is drawn down, chin is set back, eyes are squinted). These two nonmanuals are used to indicate *contrastive negation* as in (20), in which an affirmative proposition is rejected or corrected.

                                    br hs-zig
20 a   IX GOOD ALIGN, IX
        "As for him being good at putting things together, he's really not."

                                        hs-swish
    b   SMALL TOWN PREFER, BIG CITY
        "I really prefer (to live in) a small town, not in a big city."

Signed languages vary according to whether the nonmanual negative marker is required to co-occur with the negative lexical item. Languages that allow a nonmanual negative marker to either stand alone or accompany the negative lexical item are called *nonmanual dominant* (NMD); ASL and DGS (German Sign Language) are examples of these. Languages that require the use of an overt lexical negative, i.e., the nonmanual negative marker cannot stand alone, are called *manual dominant* (MD). TİD (Turkish Sign Language) and LIS (Italian Sign Language) are two such languages. In the following sections, the examples will not include the nonmanual marker as ASL allows sentences with negation to occur without them. It is for future research to determine more closely the interaction between the negative nonmanuals and negative lexical items.

4.5.2 Lexical signs for negation

We will look at four common negative items in ASL that are glossed as NOT, NEVER, NONEaltvar, and NOTHING-AT-ALL (see Figure 4.4). Traditionally, ASL linguists have treated these four items that we will discuss in this chapter as either negative adverbials or quantifiers roughly equivalent to the English words that correspond with the glosses. However, there is more to the story than that and we will see some differences in how these negatives work with ASL syntax.

4.5.2.1 NOT

NOT in ASL is basically similar in meaning and function to the corresponding English word "not". That is, it makes a whole positive predicate into a negative. Examples (21a, b) indicate that the use of NOT in ASL corresponds roughly to "not" in English. This similarity perhaps provides false assurance that negative lexical items in ASL are similar to their glosses. In the following examples, NOT occurs before the verb and has scope over the predicate.

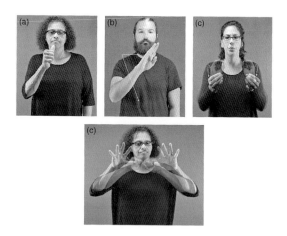

Figure 4.4 Four negative signs in ASL: (a) NOT, (b) NEVER, (c) NONE-altvar, and (d) NOTHING-AT-ALL. Images: ASL Signbank, 2018.

21 a MARY NOT LEARN ASL.
       "Mary did not learn ASL."

   b MARY NOT LEARN ASL, FRENCH.
       "Mary did not learn ASL, but French."

In (21a), we have straightforward negation of the proposition "Mary learned ASL," while in example (21b), additional information is included to show which part of the predicate is being negated.

NOT in sentence-final position does not change in meaning and exhibits much of the same behavior as preverbal NOT, showing scope over the verb phrase. Some examples of NOT in sentence-final position can be seen in (22) below.

22 a JOHN BREAK F-A-N NOT
       "John did not break the fan."

   b JOHN WATCH T-V NOT, (IX SLEEP)
       "John didn't watch TV, but he went to sleep."

However, even though NOT corresponds closely to "not" in English semantically, one important distinction is that ASL NOT can occur preverbally or clause-finally, whereas English "not" can only occur preverbally, as evidenced by the ungrammaticality of *"John broke the fan not."

We now move on to a discussion of NEVER, a sentential negative lexical item that contrasts with NOT in terms of its grammatical structure.

4.5.2.2 NEVER

NEVER is the only sign among the four discussed in this chapter that has two distinct semantic interpretations, depending on its position within the sentence. When NEVER occurs before a verb, it is quite similar to "never" in English, indicating negation of an event that takes place over time. For example, in (23b), the full interpretation of the sentence is such that John has not ever eaten fish, most likely due to lack of opportunity or availability. We show the contrast between (23a) and (23b) to better illustrate the interpretation of NEVER in preverbal position.

23   a   JOHN FINISH EAT FISH.
          "John has eaten fish."

     b   JOHN NEVER EAT FISH.
          "John has never eaten fish."

NEVER also may be positioned in the sentence-final slot. The interpretation of NEVER in sentence-final position is that the predicate is a characteristic of the subject, rather than reflecting temporal opportunities. Consider example (24). This example means that John could have eaten fish in the past or has had opportunities to eat fish, but he simply will not eat fish, possibly due to ethical concerns or allergies or whatever reason he may have.

24   JOHN EAT FISH NEVER.
      "John won't eat fish."

In sentence (25), the impossibility of Bob cooking is interpreted by his own choice or control. It is most likely that he knows how to cook or could learn how to cook but simply refuses to do so.

25   BOB COOK NEVER.
      "Bob won't/doesn't cook."

While sentence-final NEVER gives this interpretation of a characteristic of the subject, preverbal NEVER carries no such implication. The following examples illustrate that preverbal NEVER cannot have scope over the subject, but the sentence-final NEVER does.

26   a   *BOB NEVER EAT FISH, MARY IX
          "Bob will not eat fish, but Mary will."

     b   BOB EAT FISH NEVER, MARY IX
          "Bob will not eat fish, but Mary will."

The interpretation of the sentence crucially depends on where NEVER occurs. Of course, now we see that NEVER behaves quite differently than one might think from seeing the gloss for the sign, so it is important to consider carefully the error of assuming that this sign is completely analogous to "never" in English.

So far, we have discussed two sentential negative lexical items. In the next section, we will discuss two negative signs that modify noun phrases in ASL, NONEaltvar, and NOTHING-AT-ALL.

4.5.2.3 NONEaltvar and NOTHING-AT-ALL

Negative determiners have scope over nominal items, as in the "no" of "I have no paper." In English, "none" and "nothing" are *pronominal* in nature and can stand alone as in "I have seen nothing" or "She has none." In ASL, two negative lexical signs, NONEaltvar and NOTHING-AT-ALL, modify noun phrases or stand alone. Both can modify the syntactic object and typically appear in the sentence-final position. NONEaltvar can also modify the subject, but it cannot occur in the usual subject position at the beginning of a sentence and instead must occur sentence-finally. In fact, the distribution of both of these signs is even more complex, so we will not be able to describe them fully here. We provide just a few examples to illustrate their behavior.

The sentences in (27) show that NONEaltvar appears at the end of the sentence, whether it is modifying the object or the subject of the sentence.

27 a   MARY FIND <u>PAPER</u> NONEaltvar
        "Mary found no paper."

    b   SHOW-UP ON-TIME <u>INTERPRETERS</u> NONEaltvar
        "No interpreters showed up on time."

In (28), we see that NOTHING-AT-ALL[2] modifies the object and appears in sentence-final position.

28 a   STUDENT LEARN <u>ASL</u> NOTHING-AT-ALL
        "The students learned no ASL."

    b   TEACHER SEE <u>STUDENT</u> NOTHING-AT-ALL
        "The teachers saw no students."

So far, we have been concerned with the analysis of sentences that only have one overt negative lexical item. Many languages allow multiple negation, with more than one negative element in the same sentence. ASL has two different types of multiple negation: doubling and negative concord. We now move on to this topic in the next section.

4.5.3 Doubling and negative concord

ASL allows what we call *negative doubling*, as shown in (29). Sentences with double negative signs are not interpreted as positive, but emphatic. All the negative lexical items in ASL discussed in this chapter allow doubling.

29 a   MARY NONEaltvar EAT APPLE NONEaltvar
        "Mary ate no apples."

     b   **MARY NEVER EAT APPLE NEVER**
        "Mary never eats apples."

     c   **MARY NOT EAT APPLE NOT**
        "Mary did not eat the apple(s)."

There is a pragmatic effect of emphasis when doubling is used, just as we have seen before in the previous section on wh-questions.

In addition to negative doubling, ASL allows two different negative items to co-occur in the same sentence, as shown in (30). This is called negative concord and is also found in many Romance and some Germanic spoken languages. Again, the interpretation is simply negative; the two negative items do not cancel each other.

30 MARY NOT LEARN ASL NONEaltvar
     "Mary learned no ASL at all."

As we have seen in this section, the picture for negation in ASL is rather complex and dramatically different from that in English.

We have seen how scope, nonmanuals, word order, and multiple negation interact in ASL syntax. The syntactic structure for negation in ASL patterns more closely to other languages cross-linguistically than to English. What we have seen here is a brief snapshot of negation in ASL with more in-depth research to come.

4.6 Conclusion

In this chapter, a brief overview of ASL syntax has been provided, with many more components not discussed here such as pronouns, relative clauses, role-shifting, word order with agreement verbs and classifiers, eyeblinks and phrasal boundaries, rhetorical questions and wh-clefts, and the role of FINISH compared to NEVER, among others. What was discussed in this chapter was designed to provide a basic understanding of the syntactic structure of ASL, illustrating the complexity and design of word order, as reflected with stress and topicalization, nonmanual markers that interact with particular grammatical constructions, and the grammatical constructions themselves, along with wh-questions and negation. You are encouraged to find out more about these components and about what was discussed in this chapter, some of which can be found in the list for Further Reading.

Discussion questions

1   Provide two examples of instances when word order is crucial for making a distinction between two possible sentence types or interpretations.
2   ASL is a nonmanual dominant language. Does this mean ASL always uses nonmanuals for negation?
3   What do wh-questions and negation in ASL have in common?
4   Oftentimes, people have looked at ASL syntax as being simple, with little to no complexity. Why would people think that and what would be the evidence against this assumption?

Notes

1 Most of glosses are taken from ASL Signbank; the signs that corre-spond to their glosses can be viewed at https://aslsignbank.haskins.yale.edu. However, ASL Signbank is currently a work in progress, so it may not always have the gloss or translation presented in this chapter.
2 When viewing this on ASL Signbank, you will notice that their entry has the sign with both hands. It is also commonly signed with one hand.

Further reading

Petronio, K., & Lillo-Martin, D. (1997). *Wh*-movement and the position of Spec-CP. *Language, 73*(1), 18–57.
One of the first papers to discuss wh-questions in ASL, a classic in the ASL linguistics field.

Pfau, R., Steinbach, M., & Woll, B. (Eds.). (2012). *Sign language – An international handbook*. Berlin, Germany: Walter de Gruyter.
This large handbook has extensive information about the structure of different sign languages. Section C (Chapters 12–17) contains seven chapters about different areas of syntax.

Sandler, W., & Lillo-Martin, D. (2006). *Sign language and linguistic universals*. Cambridge, England: Cambridge University Press.
Even though this is much more advanced linguistics, the book has a lot of information about ASL syntax.

Zeshan, U. (2006). Negative and interrogative constructions in sign languages: a case study in sign language typology. In U. Zeshan (Ed.), *Interrogative and negative constructions in sign languages* (pp. 28–68). Nijmegen, the Netherlands: Ishara Press.
A basic cross-linguistic overview of negative constructions and questions in different sign languages is provided in this book.

References

Fischer, S.D. (1975). Influences on word order change in American Sign Language. In C. Li (Ed.), *Word order and word order change* (pp. 1–25). Austin, TX: University of Texas Press.
Liddell, S. K. 1980. *American Sign Language syntax*. The Hague, the Netherlands: Mouton.

Neidle, C., Kegl, J., MacLaughlin, D., Bahan, B., & Lee, R. G. (2000). *The syntax of American Sign Language: functional categories and hierarchical structure*. Cambridge, MA: MIT Press.

Wilbur, R. B. (1997). A prosodic/pragmatic explanation for word order variation in ASL with typological implications. In M. Vespoor, K. D. Lee & E. Sweetser (Eds.), *Lexical and syntactical constructions and the constructions of meaning* (pp. 89–104). Amsterdam, the Netherlands: John Benjamins.

Wood, S. K. (1999). *Semantic and syntactic aspects of negation in ASL.* M.A. thesis, Purdue University, West Lafayette, IN.

Chapter 5

Children with input from birth

We have seen that sign languages are complex and structured, with the same features as those found in spoken languages. We have also noted that there are some important differences between sign languages and spoken languages as a class, due to the effects of modality. We will now turn our attention to the development of sign languages in different contexts. In this chapter, we focus on the development of sign languages by Deaf children who receive fluent input from their signing parents. This context is parallel to the typical monolingual acquisition of a spoken language by hearing children. We will also include some discussion of Deaf children whose input, while beginning at birth, is in some sense degraded. And we will look at some cases of bilingualism involving a sign language and a spoken language. The following two chapters examine the development of sign languages in other contexts.

5.1 Deaf children of Deaf, signing parents

We start by considering the developmental path for Deaf children whose Deaf parents are providing them with fluent input. Fewer than 5% of Deaf children are in this situation; the vast majority are born to hearing parents who don't know any sign language when their child's hearing loss is detected. Nevertheless, it is important to start by considering this group because they constitute the baseline against which other groups might be compared.

They can be expected to show what is "typical" for sign language acquisition with full access to linguistic input from birth.

The general finding from studies of these children is that they acquire their native sign language in much the same way that hearing children acquire a spoken language. Parents and others might believe that they "teach" their child language, just as they teach their child the alphabet, counting, or words for colors and shapes. However, what parents really do is provide their child with linguistic input – they talk to their child and the child picks up, or acquires, their language (see Language in Children by Eve V. Clark in this book series). There are different styles of parenting around the world, and yet children (with few exceptions) everywhere pick up the language that is used around them naturally. This shows the importance of linguistic input, but not any particular kind of explicit teaching by parents. Learning a language is more like learning to walk; children will naturally go through stages such as crawling and standing before they walk, and while many parents may enjoy encouraging their children and helping them by holding their hands, for example, generally children will pick up walking on their own biological timetable. The same is true for language; it is acquired naturally according to a biological timetable as long as sufficient accessible input is available.

5.1.1 The first steps

Even very young infants are sensitive to the languages used around them. Experiments with hearing children have found that they notice the sounds of their language and the sound patterns of their language even right after they are born. Hearing children do receive some sound-based stimulation before they are born, so they can start to sort out the patterns of their language in the womb.

Deaf children cannot access their visual language in the womb, but they also begin to detect the linguistic patterns around them in infancy. One way we know this is by looking at the earliest linguistic productions of both sign-exposed and speech-exposed babies. Hearing babies produce pre-linguistic "babbling" which typically sounds like repeated sequences of a consonant+vowel syllable, such as "mamama", "dadada", or "googoo" by around

7–10 months of age. By 12–14 months, hearing babies' babbling is more complex and takes on the intonational patterns of the language spoken around them, so they may "sound like" they are talking even if around the same time they produce utterances containing no more than one real word. Similarly, along the same timetable children exposed to a sign language produce manual babbling parallel to the types of vocal babbling hearing children use. These manual babbles involve hand configurations and movements that could be used in a sign language, combined in novel and repetitive ways. Furthermore, the rhythm of manual babbles produced by sign-exposed babies is very different from the kinds of hand movements produced by hearing children who are not exposed to sign language. Only the manual babbles show the rhythmic qualities that match true linguistic patterns.

Researchers think that vocal and manual babbling constitute entry points into the spoken and signed linguistic systems. Babbling allows children to practice and play with the pieces of language, discovering which patterns belong to their input and how to reproduce them. It is important for deaf children to have early exposure to a sign language in part so that they can go through this process of discovery at the right time, along the way to further milestones of language development.

5.1.2 Lexical development

As babies have more and more practice with the pieces of their language, they can begin to associate particular patterns with particular meanings, and thus to learn their first words. At an average age of 10–12 months, hearing babies begin to produce their first spoken words (other than "mama" and "dada"). Researchers generally count an utterance as a "word" if it has a consistent form used with a consistent meaning; for example, "baba" might be used by a child consistently to mean "bottle," so this would count even though the child's form does not match the adult form.

When do children exposed to sign languages begin to produce their first words? There have been a number of reports that put the first signed words significantly earlier than the first spoken words – as young as eight months of age. While there is considerable variability in children's development, this two- to four-month difference in the mean would be surprising and important. The impression that children are able to learn signed words before they learn spoken words is part of the reason for the popularity of "baby signing" with hearing children. However, when looked at scientifically, there are some reasons to question this conclusion.

First, it's very important to use the same criteria for determining what is a word in speech and sign. Second, it's important to consider whether nonsigning children are producing gestures that are not considered words, while the same gestures would be considered signs for the sign-exposed children. Third, researchers also consider milestones such as a 10- or 50-word vocabulary. When such considerations are taken into account, the overall conclusion seems to be that there might be a small advantage for the first signs, due to earlier development of control over the larger muscles used to produce signs compared to speech. However, any early sign advantage (or speech disadvantage) seems to wash out when other developmental milestones are considered.

5.1.3 Phonological development

Anyone who has spent some time around young children knows that even when they begin to produce their first words, their forms are "childish." This is true for children developing a sign language as well as for children developing a spoken language. However, children's productions are not randomly different from the target; rather, they involve phonological processes invoking markedness, simplifications, and modality effects.

As discussed in Chapter 2, Phonology, signs can be described in terms of their hand configuration, location, and movement (along with additional components). As children begin to learn more and more signs, they frequently produce incorrect hand configurations. However, location errors are not as frequent, although they do exist. This contrast between hand configuration and location is found not only for children learning American Sign Language (ASL), but for other sign languages as well.

When children use an incorrect handshape, they generally replace marked configurations with unmarked ones. Recall from

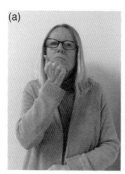 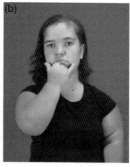

Figure 5.1 Child's production of the sign WRONG at two points in time modeled by adults: (a) age 2;00, using the incorrect handshape, and (b) age 2;03, the adult version. Image a: Copyright Diane Lillo-Martin; Image b: ASL Signbank, 2018.

Chapter 2 that the handshapes 👍, 👍, 👍, 👍, 👍, 👍, and 👍 are considered "unmarked," and can be used as the "base" hand in a two-handed asymmetrical sign such as STAND, BOTH, and MECHANIC. For children who are learning to sign, these handshapes seem easier to produce, and they may be substituted for more complex handshapes in any type of sign. For example, a two-year-old child used the 👍 handshape instead of the 👍 handshape in the signs WRONG (the child's error is demonstrated by an adult in Figure 5.1a), YELLOW, and SAME-AS. A few months later, she started producing the correct handshape (shown in Figure 5.1b), although it took a while to be completely consistent. This process is similar to substitution of simpler consonants for more complex sequences in the acquisition of English, such as saying, "tuck" instead of "truck," or "dat" for "that."

Other ways in which signing children's phonology is not yet adult-like comes from more general processes of motor development. Two examples we will discuss are proximalization and sympathy.

In order to produce the correct movement characteristic for a sign, the signer needs to know which joint to flex. As shown in Figure 5.2, the sign KNOW requires movement of the shoulder,

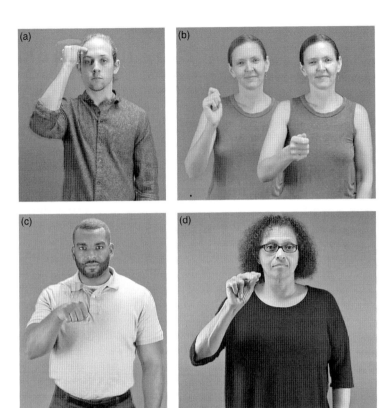

Figure 5.2 Signs that require movement of different joints: (a) KNOW, with movement at the shoulder; (b) HAMMER, with movement at the elbow; (c) YES, with movement at the wrist; and (d) NO, with movement at finger joints. Images: ASL Signbank, 2018.

HAMMER requires movement at the elbow, YES requires movement at the wrist, and NO involves movement of finger joints. When signing to a large audience, a signer might produce a sign using a joint that is closer to the body, with the result that the sign is larger and easier to see from a distance. For example, producing YES with movement of the shoulder and elbow makes it a very large sign.

For children, movement at joints that are closer – or more proximal – to the body is motorically easier than movement of the smaller, more distal joints. So, as they are learning to sign, they may proximalize signs by using joints closer to the body – ones that are not typically used to produce the sign. For example, one two-year-old produced the sign FROG with movement of the shoulder, elbow, and wrist. If you watch children's signing with this in mind, you might notice that proximalization accounts for a number of ways in which children's signing seems "loose" or "gangly" compared to adults'.

As children develop control over their bodies, they fine-tune the ability to move one hand without the other. Babies frequently move both hands up and down together; later, they can control the two arms separately more carefully. Before children have fully developed this skill they sometimes produce "sympathetic" movement of the nondominant hand while producing a sign with the dominant hand. The sympathetic movement is sometimes reduced or to the side, but the child might not yet be able to suppress it completely. For example, while signing PIG with his right hand, a child's left hand hanging at his side still moved up and down at the wrist in time with the movement of the right hand.

5.1.4 Development of morphology and syntax

When children start to produce signed words, they frequently use them to name objects (e.g., BALL), request activities (e.g., THROW), and engage in social interactions (e.g., BYE-BYE). Around the age of one year, six months (1;06), children usually start to combine words into short sentences, and these two- or three-word sentences are used alongside continued one-word utterances. When they combine words, we can ask whether their sentences are formed in the ways that the adult grammar allows, or do children break the implicit grammatical rules until they have figured them out?

We can address this question by considering the word order of simple sentences. As we saw in Chapter 4, Syntax, in ASL the underlying or "canonical" word order of a sentence is Subject–Verb–Object (SVO). As we also saw, this order can be changed by various operations such as topicalization, which can lead to the order OSV; other operations that change word order include Object Shift, which can lead to the order SOV, when the verb has special morphology for location, handling, or aspect; or Subject Pronoun Copy (SPC), which can lead to the order VOS when the subject is pronominal.

When do children seem to know the basic SVO order? Do they take a long time to learn the operations that allow word order to change? If they use orders other than SVO, do they also have appropriate morphological forms to license such changes? Some previous studies had claimed that children used a random variety of word orders, as much as 30%–40% noncanonical, but these had not carefully considered the possibility that children were making use of order-changing operations.

These questions were addressed in a study of four children's language development between the ages of 1;06 and 3;00. Once the order-changing operations were considered, it was observed that young children do tend to follow the word order varieties allowed by the adult language. Since children's utterances at this age are usually only two words long, we will consider separately the orders they use for subjects and verbs, versus verbs and objects.

This study confirmed that young children may produce a subject and a verb in either order: S V or V S. However, this study found that almost every time the V S order was used, the postverbal subject was pronominal, so this structure is adult-like according to the possibility of using SPC. For example, the children produced signed sentences such as WETneut IX "he's wet," BOY MUST IX "the boy must (do it)," or IX_1 SEARCH IX_1 "I am searching (for my shoes)." Furthermore, the proportion of pronominal subjects in preverbal position, though high, was significantly lower than that of postverbal subjects, indicating that the children are not random in their use of subjects, but following the pattern of adult ASL.

When children in this study produced OV order, usually the verb was marked for location, handling, or aspect. For example, one child signed YELLOW THROW "I threw the yellow (ball) into the corner" with location marking on the verb THROW. Another child signed CAT SEARCH[+] "I'm looking for the cat," with repetition of the verb SEARCH indicating continuous aspect. Three of the children had adult-like use of O V word order by around the age of two. The third child was more variable, and the researcher thought that this was because she was starting to use topic-like structures. However, she did not use the typical brow raise marker found in adult ASL; instead, she used a pause and/or change in the head position. We will come back to this result when we discuss another study about the development of nonmanual markers in ASL.

Overall, the results of this study show that children follow the syntactic rules for order-changing operations, and that they have acquired the morphological processes that lead to location, handling, or aspect marking.

When we consider children's development of morphological processes, we also need to discuss verb directionality, sometimes analyzed as agreement, as discussed in Chapter 3, Morphology. It has already been mentioned that children produce location marking on verbs, as in the THROW example cited earlier. What about person marking?

An early study of two deaf native signers reported that children begin to produce verb agreement around the age of two years, but that they frequently omit it and produce verbs without agreement as well. This would be similar to the common observation that children speaking English leave off verbal morphology in sentences like "he eat that." However, when the earlier study was conducted, the field had not yet discussed how to determine which verbs require agreement marking, and in which contexts. More recent views have observed that there is a relatively restricted range of contexts where adults use agreement, as discussed in Chapter 3. With this view of agreement, another study of children's development of ASL and Brazilian Sign Language (Libras) found almost no cases of missing required agreement. Most verbs that children produced were "plain," and appropriately so. This includes verbs like DRIVEsup, HAVE, and LIKE. The next highest category was verbs marked for location, such as BRING, COMEstr, and THROW. Only a small percentage of verbs required person marking, but it was produced with such verbs. Most commonly the verb GIVEo was used; an adult modeling how a child at age 1;10 produces the sign GIVOo with directionality is provided in Figure 5.3. Other signs, including FEED

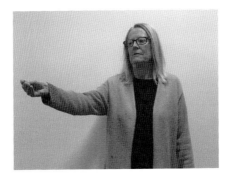

Figure 5.3 Adult modeling child's production of the sign GIVEo with directionality toward her mother at age I;I0. Image: Copyright Diane Lillo-Martin.

and SHOW, were also used with person marking by children in this study. The conclusion from this study is that children acquiring ASL may be more like children acquiring Italian, who do not omit verbal morphology very often (in contrast to children learning English, German, and French, for example).

What about other aspects of morphosyntactic development? We will summarize here studies on children's acquisition of depiction, nonmanuals, and wh-questions.

As discussed in Chapter 3, sign languages generally have a complex system for representing movement and appearance of objects and people. Initially, many researchers analyzed these constructions as involving classifiers, and they are commonly referred to as classifier constructions. More recently, some researchers use the term depiction, to emphasize the fact that the system is used to depict, iconically, what it represents, and in some cases, to move away from the classifier analysis. As in Chapter 3, we will consider this system to be a combination of morphological elements including classifiers, along with a system of depiction.

The morphological elements of this system include choosing the appropriate hand configuration for the element represented, such as using the 🖐 handshape for upright beings (people, bears), and the 🖐 handshape for vehicles (cars, bicycles). These handshapes

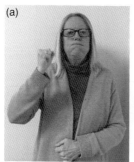 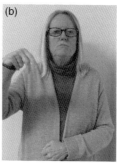

Figure 5.4 Adult modeling child's production of depicting signs with (a) DS_s 🖐 to represent pulling a train whistle and (b) DS_2 ✌ to represent a character walking. Images: Copyright Diane Lillo-Martin.

can vary across sign languages, and non-signers who might produce depicting gestures nevertheless don't typically use the sign-language-specific handshapes required. Then, it might not be surprising that children can take a number of years to get the point where they consistently use the correct handshape for each classifier. It is not uncommon for children to choose the incorrect classifier until school age.

On the other hand, children do begin using depiction at a very early age, and are able to very productively convey aspects of a referent's movement and appearance using this system. They start to incorporate it into mini storytelling and even use constructed action well (though not constructed dialogue) at a quite young age. One can find many examples in the signing of two-year-old native signers. Examples are illustrated in Figure 5.4a, where an adult models how a child of 2;02 uses a handling classifier with the 🖐 handshape to show pulling on a train whistle; and in Figure 5.4b, where she models the child's uses of the ✌ handshape at 2;06 to show the walking of a character in a book picture.

Using depiction requires using adult-like nonmanuals. At early ages, children start to use nonmanuals to express emotions, and sometimes to express the emotions of a character being referenced. However, the use of ASL grammatical nonmanuals comes in rather later. Some researchers observed that children use "hands before faces" in their development of the nonmanual markers for questions, negation, and conditionals. When there is a manual option, children use that first, and they develop the nonmanuals only later. For topics, there is no manual marker, but still, children don't seem to use the adult-like raised brows at an early age, as discussed earlier. They may only gradually develop all the pieces required for a full topic nonmanual marker, and apparently start with some kind of prosodic break.

Although children don't consistently use nonmanual markers for complex syntactic structures at an early age, they do start to use more complex varieties of sentences in the preschool years. Their earliest wh-questions tend to be one-word utterances such as, "WHAT-PU," "WHERE," and "WHY." When they produce two-word wh-questions and longer ones, they have to choose which order to use, since ASL allows multiple types of wh-questions, as discussed in Chapter 4, Syntax. Interestingly, children use a large number of wh-initial questions, such as WHAT-DO IX "What is this?" and WHERE MOTHERstr "Where's Mommy?" However, they are not limited to this position; even at the age of two years and a few months, they productively use both wh-final (GOix WHY "Why is s/he going?") and wh-double structures (WHERE RABBIT WHERE "Where is the rabbit?"). Children who are tested around the age of four preferentially use different kinds of wh-question structures depending on whether the question word is a subject, object, or adjunct (adjunct questions include "why," "how," and most "where" questions). Subject and adjunct questions overwhelmingly use the initial position, while object questions are more likely to be final (in situ). By five to six years of age, wh-double structures are much more common for adjunct questions.

5.1.5 Iconicity and sign language development

A number of researchers have been interested in whether, and if so how, iconicity affects sign language development. As we saw in Chapter 1, sign languages are nothing like mime or other purely iconic visual systems; they have grammatical structure including many "arbitrary" (non-iconic) features. However, it would be a mistake to say that there is no iconicity in sign languages, because we can observe iconicity in individual signs, in the referential system using indexical pointing, in classifiers/depiction, and in other ways. So, does iconicity make it easier to acquire aspects of sign languages?

This question has received renewed attention lately, especially in the domain of children's lexical development – their acquisition of words. It might be thought that children would find it easiest to acquire those words that are the most iconic. Several recent studies have supported this conclusion: overall, more iconic signs are more likely to be known by children in the one- to three-year-old age range, and they are learned more readily than less iconic ones. However, it should be borne in mind that this doesn't mean children don't know any non-iconic signs. Furthermore, there is some evidence (though it is mixed) that factors other than iconicity, such as phonological markedness, also play a significant role in which signs children learn earlier versus later. Also, there are various types of iconicity and different signs are iconic in different ways. Children may be more sensitive to some types of iconicity at an earlier age, and they might need to gain more real-world experience in order to even know about the iconicity of some signs. For example, the ASL sign MILK is iconically related to the action of milking a cow, but children learn the sign as an abstract word long before they know about where (cow's) milk comes from.

What about the use of iconicity in the reference system of ASL? Pointing to oneself (IX_1) functions like the pronoun "I," and pointing to the addressee (IX(addressee)) functions like the pronoun "you." Does this make it easy to acquire these signs compared to their spoken word counterparts? Children who are acquiring a spoken language sometimes mix up the reference of "I" and/or "you," something that is not so surprising when one takes into consideration that when a child hears someone say "I" it picks out that person, and when the child hears someone say "you" it picks out the child. Might children who are acquiring a sign language avoid this I/you confusion?

Studies of the acquisition of several sign languages indicate that the iconicity of pointing to self and other does not overrule the potential for confusion due to indexicality. Native signers may well produce the "I" sign to mean "you" and/or vice-versa at a young age. Like hearing/speaking children, they do not all make such mistakes and they do not necessarily consistently switch pronominal reference. However, the fact that it can happen is more evidence that children approach the language acquisition task linguistically, they learn signs as componential symbols, and they look for rules rather than relying solely on images in language.

5.2 Bimodal bilingualism

While there are some sign language users who are truly monolingual, most have some degree of bilingualism, and for some, bilingual language development takes place from birth and/or in very early childhood. For many bilingual signers, their bilingualism is *bimodal* – that is, their languages are primarily used in different modalities, sign and speech. Here we will discuss early bimodal bilingualism: first, by hearing children who acquire a sign language and a spoken language in childhood; and second, by Deaf children who use a sign language and receive a cochlear implant (CI) for learning a spoken language. Another situation fits within the description of early bilingualism, namely, Deaf children who use more than one sign language (for example, ASL and Japanese Sign Language). However, there are no published studies that we know of with this population, although such research is just getting started. As for signers learning the written version of a spoken language in school, and later learners of a second language, including a second sign language, or a sign language as a second language in a second modality, these contexts will be discussed in Chapter 6.

5.2.1 Simultaneous acquisition of a sign language and a spoken language – Kodas

While the percent of Deaf children who grow up with signing parents is very low, there are a good number of hearing children with Deaf, signing parents. These children are exposed to a sign language from birth, and they generally have plenty of access to spoken language input, so they may grow up as bimodal bilinguals.

As noted in Chapter 1, hearing adult children of Deaf adults are often referred to as Codas; we will use the variant Kodas to indicate our current focus on "kids."

In any community where the home language is different from the dominant language of the community, children learning these two languages may be relatively balanced simultaneous bilinguals, or they might experience a plateau in development of their "heritage" language, the home language. Often, the home language is reserved for home and family activities, and when school takes over a larger proportion of a child's life, the child will tend to favor the language used at school, in the community, and especially by peers. Nevertheless they may maintain conversational fluency in their home language and in many cases they function bilingually as adults.

The same can be said for children who are growing up as bimodal bilinguals. At young ages, they may be dominant in the sign language used at home, but they generally pick up the spoken language of the community and often it becomes the language they use the most, even if the home language continues to hold a special connection. We can consider how children manage with two languages during the period of language acquisition, including questions about how children manage to "separate" their languages, and how they allow them to interact.

Many people who are not researchers might wonder how a very young child who is exposed to two spoken languages can keep the languages apart. How does the child know that "cat" belongs to English and "gato" belongs to Spanish? On the other hand, separating the two language inputs might be much easier for children acquiring a sign language and a spoken language, since the words of one are signed and the words of the other are spoken! While it is true that the task seems to be much simpler for bimodal bilinguals, in fact it turns out that even children learning two spoken languages do not have much trouble knowing which language is which. From an early age both kinds of bilingual children learn vocabulary in both languages, and they tend to use the appropriate language with (monolingual) speakers of one language or the other – though they do persist in using the "wrong" language sometimes, including hearing children using speech with their Deaf parents, knowing that communication often does take place because the Deaf adults are skilled at interacting with people who don't know their language well.

Like unimodal bilinguals, bimodal bilinguals also have opportunities to allow their languages to interact. Sometimes, a language feature that has been acquired in one language will "influence" the other language, so that children will use that feature even if the second language doesn't work the same way. For example, Chinese–English bilingual children might follow the dominant Chinese structure for forming wh-questions, leaving the wh-word *in situ*, even in English, where that structure is only used in certain contexts (see Chapter 4). However, language "mixing" is also used by bilingual adults in rule-governed, creative ways, for purposes that include marking of in-group status with other bilinguals. For example, speakers may code-switch between their languages, substituting words or phrases from one language and mixing them quite fluently. Although some people frown on such practices, in fact they follow grammatical rules and indicate a high degree of proficiency.

For bimodal bilinguals, code-blending is used rather than code-switching for the same kinds of functions. Code-blending involves simultaneous production of parts of an utterance in speech and sign. It is different from "simultaneous communication," or "SimCom," a method invented for representing English on the hands in deaf education. SimCom necessarily follows English word order and also preferably includes a separate sign for each word. Code-blending can use ASL word order in both languages, or even in limited cases use an ASL structure together with an English structure. For example, code-blending can combine an ASL classifier with an English verb phrase, as shown below. The box indicates that the parts of the utterance inside the box are produced at the same time.

ASL: | DS_2(walk-around) |
English: He | walked around |

Code-blending is an opportunity for bilinguals chatting with each other to employ both of their languages in creative ways. It seems that the grammatical patterns of code-blending are similar to those of code-switching, but further work on this topic is currently in progress.

5.2.2 Simultaneous acquisition of a sign language and a spoken language: DDCI

Hearing children in signing families are not the only children growing up as bimodal bilinguals. Some Deaf children in Deaf, signing families receive a CI at a young age. A CI is a device that is surgically inserted to provide stimulation to the auditory nerve. A person with a CI does not hear the same way that people who have a functioning cochlea hear, and children with CIs must go through speech training to learn how to use their CI to perceive speech and produce it. When Deaf children receive a CI, some of them do learn to use spoken language at levels that eventually correspond to their typically hearing age-mates, although there is a great deal of variability in outcomes and some children do not catch up in their spoken language abilities. What happens if a child is implanted and is taught to use spoken language while at the same time they use sign language at home?

While it is a small population, there have been some studies of children in this unique situation, whom we refer to as DDCI (Deaf children with Deaf parents, using a CI). The studies of this group reveal that they are in many ways very similar to Kodas, once they have had enough time to start to use spoken language with the CI. For example, by the age of around five, DDCIs and Kodas perform very similarly on standard tests of ASL and spoken English (at the right levels for their chronological age). Analyses of their spoken language indicate that at relatively early stages of development they make the same kinds of "errors" in as typically developing children, such as leaving off verb inflections or articles (like "the" and "a/an"). These studies indicate that the use of sign language does not interfere with children's development of spoken language, and it may even help. However, it is not known yet whether results would be similar for Deaf children whose hearing parents are learning to sign with them.

5.3 Effects of non-native input

Our focus in this chapter has been on sign language development by Deaf children who receive input in a sign language from birth. While this population is rather small, only a relatively small proportion of that population receives input from parents who themselves had input from birth – they would be third-generation Deaf or higher. In fact, most studies do not distinguish between Deaf signing parents who were themselves native signers and those who were not. However, we know that if a Deaf child is not exposed to sign language until the age of five years or later, there can be long-lasting effects of delayed exposure; this will be discussed in some detail in Chapter 6. One study focused on a seven-year-old Deaf child (Simon) whose only input in ASL came from parents who themselves were rather late signers, and lacked some of the complex elements of ASL grammar. What happens in that context?

The study focused on the use of ASL classifiers, also known as depicting signs, as discussed in Chapter 3. This structure was chosen because it was already known that Deaf signers with late exposure do not perform like native signers with these complex elements, but rather omit some of the required pieces when tested on production. As expected the parents performed like other adults who had been late learners, and below the ceiling level of performance by adult native signers. On the other hand, Simon himself performed like native signing age-mates, well above his parents, on almost all components of the same test.

These results indicate that even if the parents show effects of being late learners, their child can "regularize" the imperfect input. This is considered to be one of the reasons why young children are generally better language learners than adults – they have the ability to organize their input and find the inherent rules and patterns in it. In fact, they often "over-regularize" by applying a rule to cases that for the adult are exceptional. This is why young English-speaking children say "goed" and "foots." Their application of the regular rule even where the adult would use an exception makes the children temporarily sound non-adult in the English case. However, the ability to form rules even if the input is irregular gives Simon and children like him a real advantage.

5.4 Conclusion

Overall, we see that Deaf children with input in a sign language from birth can acquire it along a timetable that is very similar to that followed by hearing children learning a spoken language. The

100 Children with input from birth

fact that a sign language is produced by the hands may lend a slight advantage to signing children, since they are able to produce recognizable words somewhat earlier than speaking children can. They progress through stages including growing their vocabulary, beginning to produce two-word utterances, and expanding in morphology and syntax. It should not be surprising that sign languages are acquired as natural human languages, but it is an important point.

Furthermore, if children are exposed to both a sign language and a spoken language, they are able to become fully bilingual. Their use of one language need not interfere with their development of the other, and like other bilinguals, they find that each is used in its appropriate contexts and purposes.

However, only a very small proportion of Deaf children are exposed to sign language input from birth. How language develops in contexts of later exposure is the topic of the next chapter.

Discussion questions

1 When a Deaf child is born to Deaf, signing parents, what is special about the way they acquire language?
2 What kinds of "errors" do children make when they acquire a language? Do children acquiring a sign language make the same kinds of errors?
3 What are the ways that children can be bilingual using a sign language as one of their languages? Does bilingualism hurt children's mastery of language?
4 Is a sign language easier to acquire than a spoken language? Why or why not? Defend your answer against those who might disagree.
5 If parents use a sign language regularly but they did not learn it as their first language, how is this likely to affect the way their child learns to sign?

Further reading

Chen Pichler, D. (2012). Acquisition. In R. Pfau, M. Steinbach, & B. Woll (Eds.), *Sign language: an international handbook* (pp. 647–686). Berlin, Germany: Walter de Gruyter.
This article provides a comprehensive overview of research on sign language acquisition.

Chen Pichler, D., Kuntze, M., Lillo-Martin, D., Quadros, R. M. de, & Stumpf, M. R. (2018). *Sign language acquisition by deaf and hearing children: a bilingual introduction.* Washington, DC: Gallaudet University Press.

This text is all in ASL, with bulleted text slides accompanying the signing and a spoken English voiceover. It overviews key concepts about sign language acquisition, including native signers, those with delayed/degraded input, and bimodal bilinguals.

Chen Pichler, D., Lee, J., & Lillo-Martin, D. (2014). Language development in ASL-English bimodal bilinguals. In D. Quinto-Pozos (Ed.), *Multilingual aspects of signed language communication and disorder* (pp. 235–260). Bristol, England: Multilingual Matters.

This chapter is an overview of sign and spoken language development by Kodas.

Lillo-Martin, D. (2016). Sign language acquisition studies. In E. L. Bavin & L. R. Naigles (Eds.), *The Cambridge handbook of child language* (2nd Ed., pp. 504–526). Cambridge, England: Cambridge University Press.

This chapter provides a summary of much previous research on sign language acquisition, organized according to the research themes each study addresses.

Bibliography

Chamberlain, C., Morford, J. P., & Mayberry, R. I. (2000). *Language acquisition by eye.* Mahwah, NJ: Lawrence Erlbaum Associates.

Davidson, K., Lillo-Martin, D., & Chen Pichler, D. (2014). Spoken English language development among native signing children with cochlear implants. *Journal of Deaf Studies and Deaf Education, 19*(2), 238–250.

Lillo-Martin, D. (2016). Sign language acquisition studies. In E. L. Bavin & L. R. Naigles (Eds.), *The Cambridge handbook of child language* (2nd Ed., pp. 504–526). Cambridge, England: Cambridge University Press.

McIntire, M. (1977). The acquisition of ASL hand configurations. *Sign Language Studies, 16,* 247–260.

Meier, R. P. (2002). The acquisition of verb agreement: pointing out arguments for the linguistic status of agreement in signed languages. In G. Morgan & B. Woll (Eds.), *Current developments in the study of signed language acquisition.* Amsterdam, the Netherlands: John Benjamins.

Meier, R. P., & Newport, E. L. (1990). Out of the hands of babes: on a possible sign advantage in language acquisition. *Language, 66*, 1–23.

Newport, E. L., & Meier, R. P. (1985). The acquisition of American Sign Language. In D. I. Slobin (Ed.), *The cross-linguistic study of language acquisition* (pp. 881–938). Hillsdale, NJ: Lawrence Erlbaum Associates.

Petitto, L. A. (1987). On the autonomy of language and gesture: evidence from the acquisition of personal pronouns in American Sign Language. *Cognition, 27*(1), 1–52.

Singleton, J. L., & Newport, E. L. (2004). When learners surpass their models: the acquisition of American Sign Language from inconsistent input. *Cognitive Psychology, 49*(4), 370–407.

Chapter 6

Contexts of later language development

In Chapter 5, we discussed the acquisition of a sign language in contexts where children have access to linguistic input from birth, focusing on Deaf children with Deaf, fluent signing parents, and hearing children of Deaf signing parents (Kodas). However, these contexts are relatively infrequent; most Deaf children who acquire a sign language have hearing parents who had no knowledge of sign before their Deaf child was born. Often, these children eventually do use a sign language and it becomes their primary language, but there may be long-lasting effects of their early period without accessible language input. In this chapter we examine sign language development under such circumstances, starting with studies of children and young people, followed by studies with adults who were tested decades after they began signing. The intriguing question of what happens before such children begin receiving accessible input – or if they continue into adulthood without input in a natural sign language – will be discussed in the next chapter on homesigners.

One additional context of later sign language development will also be discussed in the current chapter: adults who are learning a sign language as a second language when their first language was spoken (there is not yet enough research to report on patterns of second sign language learning by adults who already know one sign language). While relatively less research has addressed this population, we will bring up a few findings that have emerged and mention areas for future studies. Finally, we will briefly review some research on the learning of the written version of a spoken language by Deaf signers.

6.1 The critical period hypothesis

It is important to set the stage for this chapter by reviewing a hypothesis about language development that has been very influential and important. It is often observed that young children are much better language learners than adults are. Children can even pick up multiple languages with ease, as long as there is sufficient accessible input and others to use the languages with. In addition, if children experience a brain injury that affects their language, they seem to be better at regaining linguistic abilities than are adults who have a similar experience. On the basis of such observations, it has been hypothesized that there is a "critical period," or a special window of opportunity, during which language can be acquired easily. After the critical period is over, language development becomes more difficult, possibly because different mental resources must be used.

While this hypothesis is well known, there are many questions about some of the details. For example, is the end of the critical period at puberty, as some have claimed, or does it actually close much earlier? Is there a difference between learning a first language versus learning a second language after the critical period? And since language learning after the critical period does not seem to be impossible (at least in most cases), what part of the language acquisition process does the critical period actually affect?

It is impossible to fully address these questions if the only data come from hearing people learning spoken languages. A scientist would want to test the hypothesis by withholding language input from children until they reach different ages, to see how their language develops after one, three, five, or ten years of deprivation (for example). However, this would be unethical, and it is fortunately almost never the case that a hearing child is naturally completely cut off from linguistic input. Sadly, this situation is common for Deaf children: if they cannot access the spoken language used around them and there is no one providing input in a natural sign language, the "experiment of nature" can be run. What happens to first-language acquisition when accessible input is delayed? Does it make a difference if the child begins to sign after a few years or in the teens? And how long are any effects observed? These questions have been addressed by studies of Deaf learners, to which we turn now, starting with studies of children/youth in Section 6.2, and moving to studies of adults in Section 6.3.

6.2 Children receiving late input in a sign language

There are many studies that compare results on American Sign Language (ASL) tests for native signers (with input from birth) versus non-native signers (whose input begins at various ages). These studies generally find that native signers score better on tests of ASL, and even on tests of English, academic achievement, social development, etc.

We know of only one project that gathered intensive data about the process of sign language development after a period of delay of about five years. Mei and Cal are two unrelated students who started attending a school for the Deaf around the same time at the age of five to six, having had essentially no accessible linguistic input previously (although there was a service provider who worked with one of them, this person knew only a few signs). Both were assessed as knowing only a few signs (less than 25) at the time they entered the school. The school, a residential facility, employed a Deaf adult to serve as a language model with the children, so they were immersed in ASL once they started attending, though there were long gaps during vacations and other periods. A researcher began to video record the children on a regular basis shortly after they started at the school, continuing to record them for four years. This intensive data set served as the basis for a series of studies that focused on aspects of language that were expected to be most affected by the delayed exposure.

The first finding from this study is that after they started their immersion in ASL, the two children progressed through similar stages of language development as native signing Deaf children, though much later, of course. For example, they started by using one-sign utterances, and progressed to a two-sign stage. During the two-sign stage, their signing was a lot like that of two-year-olds, except for one thing: since they were much older, they tried to convey more sophisticated concepts than a two-year-old would do. For example, their utterances expressed typically late-appearing semantic relations such as intention (FUTUREstr LEAVEo "S/he will leave") and recurrence (ALWAYS SNEEZE "S/he always sneezes"). This finding indicates that the progression through early stages (such as the two-word stage) observed in native signers and children learning spoken languages seems to be a part of language development in particular, not due to a very general stage of cognitive development that would characterize two-year-olds.

At that two-word stage, what do children's sentences look like? As we mentioned in Chapter 5, Deaf children with Deaf, signing parents productively employ both the default word orders of ASL, Subject Verb and Verb Object, and also alternative orders as licensed by grammatical properties of particular sentences, resulting in Verb Subject and Object Verb. The children with delayed linguistic input did not follow the same pattern. Instead, they used mainly S V and V O word orders and failed to take advantage of the alternative orders possible. It's possible that they learned to make use of these word orders later. However, since some of the O V orders are contingent on the appropriate use of ASL's morphological markers, it is also possible that the later learners had not yet developed those morphological elements, explaining their delayed acquisition. The final, most extensive study of this project focuses on the development of morphology.

As we showed in Chapter 3, Morphology, ASL has an extensive system that uses the directionality of verb sign movement to indicate the people and/or locations of events. In Chapter 5, we saw that Deaf children with native input in ASL begin to use this system appropriately around two to three years of age. There may be some errors, particularly errors of omission, at the beginning stages, but children are productively producing both person and location marking relatively early. This was not the case for Mei and Cal. They used the spatial verbs, indicating the location of events, relatively well, and maintained a high level of accuracy in their usage of this marking over time. However, they omitted verb directionality for person agreement frequently, and they never improved to a high proportion of correct usage in obligatory contexts – even after four years of immersion, when they were around ten years old. Since they achieved the two-word stage rather quickly after their immersion, it is almost like they spent at least four years trying to learn something that native signers achieve within one year, at least within this very specific domain.

The contrast between directionality for person and location marking is striking. It is an indication that the special effects of late acquisition are very fine-tuned. It will take more research to determine exactly what domains of language are most severely affected, but these results, together with those with adults to be discussed in Section 6.3, indicate that the critical period is not a blunt instrument.

There are two projects that have examined teenagers with delayed sign language input. These children from hearing families had various reasons for their delayed linguistic input, both spoken and signed, but eventually they were placed in a school or program for the Deaf that used ASL, where their immersion began. In the first study, two adolescents were immersed in ASL in their early teens. Their sign production was observed, recorded, and analyzed five times each over a period of about 2½ years. At the first observation, neither participant used ASL agreement forms or classifiers. During the observation period, they started using classifiers and eventually they used directionality, but it did not reach 100% accuracy. It is not reported whether they used person versus location marking differentially.

The same participants from this production study were tested for comprehension after seven years of exposure to ASL. When asked to choose a picture matching a signed sentence they viewed once at normal speed, they responded only slightly above chance level. When they were allowed to view the signed sentences multiple times, their scores increased. Thus, it seems that their delayed linguistic exposure affected their language development such that they still showed processing load effects even after seven years of experience.

A more recent project has conducted multiple studies with three Deaf adolescents who began exposure to ASL in their teens, with the pseudonyms Shawna, Cody, and Carlos. When assessed at 12–24 months post exposure, the three teens all showed ASL vocabulary knowledge above the level for Deaf native signers at ages corresponding to their length of exposure. This indicates that once they were immersed, they were able to learn ASL signs relatively quickly. However, like Mei and Cal, their average sentence length was around (just over) two signs. So, it is even more clear that language development needs to proceed through a two-sign stage (of some sort), whether it takes place while a child is two years old or older, and regardless of a possible larger overall vocabulary size.

Two of the three adolescents (Shawna and Carlos) also participated in a study that used magnetoencephalography, a method for determining which brain regions are involved in cognitive tasks. This study found that both late learners used very different areas of the brain for processing recently learned signs, in comparison to native Deaf signers and even hearing people who have been learning ASL as a second language for the same length of time as Shawna and Carlos used it as a first language. This result provides striking evidence that late exposure to a first language does affect the way it is acquired and processed in the brain, even in a linguistic domain where later learning seems more straightforward (learning new words).

6.3 Adults who had received late input in a sign language

A number of studies have examined the ASL used by Deaf adults for whom it is a primary language, but who began their exposure to ASL late. These studies typically find that some aspects of grammatical development have been negatively affected by the delay in language exposure. In some cases, no differences are found in the linguistic behavior, but there are evidently processing effects such that later learners do not show the same kind of deep, rapid language processing that native signers do.

For example, in one study, adults who had been using ASL for decades were tested on their knowledge of ASL syntax and morphology. One group were native signers, another group had begun their exposure to ASL around five years of age, and the third group was exposed to ASL only around age 13. Before their exposure to ASL, these people had been in oral educational programs, but their development of spoken language was limited.

The study found that the adults did not have difficulty with understanding the basic Subject Verb Object word order of ASL. However, their production and comprehension of morphological components including verb agreement and verbs of motion and location (classifiers / depicting signs, as discussed in Chapter 3) was indeed affected by their age of exposure. Those with native exposure scored almost perfectly on the tests, although there was some variability. Those with exposure starting around five performed notably lower, and those whose exposure began at 13 scored even worse. Thus, this study shows that the age of exposure can affect grammatical knowledge even for signers who use ASL as a primary language for many years.

Additional studies have looked at this issue in more depth. One study compared Deaf people of about the same ages, when one group had delayed first-language (L1) acquisition of sign language, and the other were people who were born hearing and learned spoken language but became Deaf and learned sign language later in life, as a second language (L2). When both groups were tested on an ASL sentence recall task, the late L2 signers performed significantly better than the late L1 signers did, producing sentences that were grammatical and semantically related to the target sentence much more often. A similar result was found using a grammaticality judgment task. L2 signers who became Deaf later in life were more accurate at detecting ungrammatical sentences in ASL than were those Deaf signers who were late L1 learners. As would be expected, the native signers performed the best on these tests.

Research has shown notable effects of late learning on the processing of sign language. For example, one study looked at phonological processing by having participants "shadow" a video of signing – they were asked to repeat back the signs they saw immediately as they occurred, without even waiting until the end of a sentence. The researchers found that native signers performed fairly well, but when they made mistakes, they might substitute a sign that had a similar meaning to the target sign. This indicates that the participants are fully processing the input and getting to the meaning, despite the very quick response required. On the other hand, late L1 signers more often make phonological errors; that is, they produce a sign that looks like the target sign but is different from it on one parameter (cf. Chapter 2). This results in a sign whose meaning is completely different, and incorrect for the context. Such a pattern indicates that the signers are not processing the sentences quickly, and they are repeating signs back without reaching meaning.

In other tests, later L1 learners might make phonological-based mistakes by choosing a response that is related to the proper response based on form. On the flip side, some researchers have observed that later learners may produce signs with an accent, where their sign production is not quite like native signers, especially when it comes to rhythm and prosody. These kinds of results also indicate that later learners are slower processors, and may spend more time on the phonological level, taking more time to get to the meaning of a sentence.

In ordinary conversation, these effects are not likely to interfere greatly. Later learners can use ASL as their primary language quite effectively. However, they may take just a bit longer to process than native signers, and this can have effects in other domains. For example, numerous studies have found that native signers perform better academically than later learners. Delayed linguistic input can affect cognitive development and social/emotional development as well.

A recent study looked at children attending schools for the Deaf employing a bilingual approach, where ASL is taught early and is used as the language of instruction (at least for some subjects). In this context, children with hearing parents who entered the school early were more likely to score at levels comparable to the native signers on tests looking at language skills such as analogy and reasoning. That is, with early entry to a sign-rich environment, Deaf children of hearing parents performed better. On the other hand, many Deaf children enter schools using sign language only after some years of trying (unsuccessfully) a mainstream approach with hearing technology, such as hearing aids or cochlear implants. In this context, late sign language acquisition effects are very strong, and the students may perform poorly on both sign language and spoken language assessments. There are therefore many reasons to think that better outcomes are most likely to be associated with early exposure to a full sign language, and the earlier the better.

6.4 Adults learning a sign language as L2

Researchers have begun to study the ways that nonsigning adults learn a sign language as a second (or additional) language. Because these adults are learning a new language (L2) in a new modality (M2), sometimes they are referred to as M2L2 learners. We know many of the ways that knowledge of a first spoken language affects the learning of a second spoken language. But is it different when the first language is spoken and the second is signed?

Second language learning is different from first-language acquisition in several ways. In the first place, the L2 learner has an L1 for comparison, and often some grammatical pieces from L1 will show up in L2 until the learner is more fluent in L2. This is known as "transfer," and while it is usually discussed as a negative factor (when the L1 aspect is not part of L2), it can also be facilitative. For spoken language M1L2 learners, transfer can occur with phonological and morphosyntactic grammatical elements.

For M2L2 learners, can transfer occur at the phonological level? It might be considered impossible, since the articulatory mechanisms of speech and sign are so different. However, at least one study has found evidence for such transfer. This study started from the premise that speakers also use gestures, including some that are relatively conventionalized and have a consistent use/interpretation. Such gestures include the fist-shaking "yes!" and the gesture to mean "call me" using a form similar to the ASL sign for TELEPHONE. Although the gestures are conventionalized, there is considerable variability in the details of their form. The researchers wondered whether features of these known gestures would creep into the learning of real signs.

The researchers recruited hearing nonsigners before they started learning ASL. They were asked to repeat gestures and signs that were shown on video. Then the researchers did very detailed coding of the handshapes used for both gestures and signs. What they found revealed that novice sign learners are indeed influenced by their previous knowledge of gesture, but this effect is also subject to linguistic constraints. For very unmarked handshapes, the use of a slightly different form in gesture could carry over to a previously unknown sign. For example, a participant who produced the "yes" gesture using an ✊ handshape rather than the modeled 🤚 handshape also produced the sign for SYMBOL using the nontarget 🤚 handshape.

What about other areas of sign language learning? One study looked at the ways that learners (of Catalan Sign Language, LSC) used full noun phrases, pronouns, and null elements in their signed discourse. Typically, native signers would use a full noun phrase to introduce a new referent, and they would use a null element for reference maintenance, since LSC is a language that allows this kind of structure (as is ASL). However, language learners in many spoken languages have a tendency to overuse overt forms, such as overt pronouns or full noun phrases where a null element is permitted. Similarly, the LSC learners overused overt pronouns. Note that the spoken language Catalan, which these learners all knew, also permits null elements in the same contexts, so the learners did not simply transfer their knowledge from Catalan. Instead, there seems to be a general tendency for over-specification by learners, and this applies to sign language learners just as it does for spoken language L2 learners.

Other studies of sign language M2L2 learners are currently underway, examining the kinds of effects that might be expected due to language transfer, but potentially complicated by the differences in modality. It remains to be seen whether, and if so, in what ways, learning a sign language as an L2 differs from learning a spoken language as an L2.

6.5 Signers learning the written form of a spoken language

Although it is not about sign language acquisition, we will briefly summarize here some research on the learning of a spoken language (in its written form) by Deaf signers. Given that the signers may show evidence of transfer from their first language, sign language is indeed relevant in this context.

In general, there are many studies that find an effect of age of sign language acquisition on competency in learning the written version of a spoken language. Those signers with a strong foundation of skills in the L1 generally perform better on written language assessments than later L1 signers do. This finding is taken to reinforce the need for a strong L1 foundation even when the spoken/written language is a goal.

Such results are not to say that there is no influence from the first language on the learning of the second. To the contrary, it must be said that sometimes ASL structures can find their way into the written forms used by Deaf signers. For example, Deaf writers may omit elements that are not used or are optional in ASL, even if they are obligatory in English, such as articles (a, the), pronominal subjects, and verbal morphology. In this, however, they are not unique – these kinds of uses are common to others who are learning English as an L2. In fact, there are many parallels in English competence between Deaf readers and hearing English L2 readers, when this possibility is considered and tested. Thus, it is appropriate to consider the kinds of L2 teaching approaches that are used with hearing learners as potentially useful for Deaf readers.

Other parallels between Deaf readers and hearing bilinguals have also been demonstrated. Researchers investigating bilingual processing have found evidence that both languages are active in a bilingual even in contexts that only require one language. The connections between languages in a bilingual's brain simply stay active all the time. The same is true for Deaf readers who are bilingual in a sign language and (the written form of) a spoken language. They show the kinds of processing effects in lexical access and other experiments that indicate continued activation of both their languages. Hearing bimodal bilinguals also show these effects. Overall, it is clear that the way the brain processes a spoken language and a sign language are similar enough that bilingual effects observed in two spoken languages also carry over to other contexts.

6.6 Conclusion

This chapter has focused on contexts of language development where exposure begins later than birth: those Deaf children who experience a period of delay before accessible linguistic input is available; L2 learners of a sign language; and Deaf signers' learning of a written language. While the view of a critical period that ends sharply at puberty is no longer maintained, it is clear that any delay of linguistic input can affect a child's language development, and in turn their development in many areas. The most important take-home message from these observations should be that early exposure to accessible linguistic input is vital for the development of Deaf children.

However, both L1 and L2 learners frequently pick up some parts of a language later in life. Researchers are still trying to determine which aspects of language are more likely to be acquired in such contexts, and which ones are more fragile. There are numerous indications that verbal morphology and other functional elements are less likely to be thoroughly learned, and while basic syntactic structures are learnable, more complex ones can pose a significant challenge. Phonology is among the most difficult aspects for late acquisition, which is why late learners of many types typically display an accent. On the other hand, vocabulary can be learned later in life, and indeed, even first-language speakers or signers continue to pick up new words over their lifetime.

Although our discussion has focused on sign language acquisition after late exposure, what happens before this later exposure begins? If Deaf children are not able to access spoken language and are not addressed using a sign language, do they completely lack any linguistic elements? A series of studies has determined that no, in this context Deaf children innovate their own communicative system, known as Homesign. In the next chapter, we discuss aspects of Homesign as used by Deaf individuals, and what happens to a homesign system when Deaf individuals form a community.

Discussion questions

1   What is one area of language that is negatively affected by delayed linguistic exposure?

2   Is the critical period hypothesis supported, contradicted, or refined by research on signers? Give evidence for your position.

3   If you were an adult trying to learn a sign language as a second language, what could you do to enhance your learning based on what research says?

4   Discuss the ways that children are able to go beyond the input they have received, and the limits on this ability. What are the consequences for situations in which children lack access to a language in their early years?

Further reading

Berk, S., & Lillo-Martin, D. (2012). The two-word stage: motivated by linguistic or cognitive constraints? *Cognitive Psychology*, *65*, 118–140.
This is one of the papers discussed in the text about children with delayed exposure to ASL (Mei and Cal).

Chen Pichler, D., & Koulidobrova, E. (2016). Acquisition of sign language as a second language (L2). In M. Marschark, & P.E. Spencer (Eds.), *The Oxford handbook of deaf studies in language: research, policy, and practice* (pp. 218–230). Oxford, England: Oxford University Press.
This paper provides an overview of L2 sign language learning.

Mayberry, R. (2010). Early language acquisition and adult language ability: what sign language reveals about the critical period for language. In M. Marschark & P.E. Spencer (Eds.), *The Oxford handbook of deaf studies, language, and education* (Vol. 2, pp. 281–291). Oxford, England: Oxford University Press.
This chapter is a nice summary of a number of papers looking at critical period effects in late L1 signers.

Morford, J. P. (2003). Grammatical development in adolescent first-language learners. *Linguistics*, *41*(4), 681–721.
This article discusses late sign language development in Deaf adolescents.

Morford, J. P., & Mayberry, R. I. (2000). A reexamination of "early exposure" and its implications for language acquisition by eye. In C. Chamberlain, J. P. Morford, & R. I. Mayberry (Eds.), *Language acquisition by eye* (pp. 111–127). Hillsdale, NJ: Lawrence Erlbaum Associates.
This chapter provides a hypothesis about why early linguistic exposure is so crucial for language development.

Newport, E. L. (1990) Maturational constraints on language learning. *Cognitive Science*, *14*, 11–28.
This article presents some information about a large-scale study of Deaf adults with exposure at different ages, and how the results from such a study fit in with the critical period hypothesis.

Ormel, E., Hermans, D., Knoors, H., & Verhoeven, L. (2012). Cross-language effects in written word recognition: the case of bilingual deaf children. *Bilingualism: Language and Cognition, 15*(2), 280–303. This is one of several papers that show bilingual effects for Deaf readers.

Bibliography

Ferjan Ramírez, N., Lieberman, A.M., & Mayberry, R.I. (2013). The initial stages of firstlanguage acquisition begun in adolescence: when late looks early. *Journal of Child Language, 40*, 391–414.

Henner, J., Caldwell-Harris, C.L., Novogrodsky, R., & Hoffmeister, R. (2016). American Sign Language syntax and analogical reasoning skills are influenced by early acquisition and age of entry to signing schools for the deaf. *Frontiers in Psychology, 7*, article 1982. doi: 10.3389/fpsyg.2016.01982

Mayberry, R. I., & Eichen, E. B. (1991). The long-lasting advantage of learning sign language in childhood: another look at the critical period for language acquisition. *Journal of Memory and Language, 30*(4), 486–512.

Chapter 7

Homesign systems

In this chapter, we will consider homesign systems, which are self-generated linguistic systems created by Deaf children. Some of these Deaf children who use homesigns go on to school, leaving behind this system of communication, but there are others who continue to use their homesign system as adults. We will look at a few basic characteristics of homesign systems in both young and adult homesigners.

7.1 Introduction

All humans use gestures to communicate with each other to some extent, but most gestures are used to support speech rather than being used as a separate system of communication. The meaning of conventional gestures is generally designated by the community at large. For instance, the "OK" gesture in which the forefinger meets the thumb in a small circular shape is well-attested in the United States as meaning "okay" or "all good," but in Brazil, Germany, or Russia, this gesture is considered vulgar as it refers to a private orifice on the body. Many times, humans will point to an object to indicate what they are talking about, what they want, or to show where something is. Signed languages not only incorporate these meanings for the indexical point but also use it as a pronoun meaning "she," "he," "it" or as a demonstrative "this." As we have seen in Chapters 2–4, signed languages use a manual component as the basis for their linguistic system that is complex in phonology, morphology, and syntax. Moreover, as discussed in Chapter 5, children typically learn signed languages such as American Sign Language (ASL), Russian Sign Language, Japanese Sign Language, or Brazilian Sign Language (Libras), from a source language provided by their parents or from school.

Homesigned systems are linguistic systems based on gestures produced by Deaf people with little to no input from a source language. In every country in the world, there are homesigners, both young and adult, whose linguistic system of communication is self-generated, using innate tools for language creation. Research by anthropologists and linguists have unearthed homesign systems all over the world in remote parts of countries such as Australia, Bangladesh, Belgium, Brazil, Britain, Canada, China, Guatemala, Iran, Japan, Mauritius, Mexico, the Netherlands, Nicaragua, Papua New Guinea, Rennell Islands, Taiwan, Turkey, the United States, and the West Indies. Not only that, many, if not most, Deaf children start out as homesigners for the first few years of their lives (before they go to school) because they have limited exposure to the spoken language used in their family or the sign language of the Deaf community. As we have discussed in Chapter 6, 95% of Deaf children have hearing parents, most of whom do not use sign language with their children. These children then learn a sign language (or a spoken language) as a late first language with consequent deficits in their phonology, morphology, and syntax because they did not have the necessary early exposure to the target language. In order to communicate with those around them, these children sometimes use homesigns which are usually abandoned once the child is exposed to a full language.

7.2 What are homesigns?

Homesigns are gestural components of a self-generated linguistic system used for communication by Deaf children who have no or little accessible exposure to another existing language, signed or spoken. There are some differences in the syntactic, phonological, and morphological structure of a given homesign system compared to a fully established language. Much of the existing and current research on homesign systems focuses on these aspects of language to better understand how language is created or arises from a small set of linguistic constructs. We cannot artificially create an experiment in which we withhold language from children to investigate what happens when children have to figure out ways to communicate on their own. However, we can use "experiments of nature" in which this naturally arises without any human interference. Looking into how a homesign linguistic system is constructed and which components of language are included in said system provides us with a window into the human brain and how it creates language. The rest of the chapter will discuss these components in more detail.

For a homesign system to appear as a mode of communication by a Deaf child, certain environmental conditions must be met. Different cases of homesign systems tend to share the same characteristics. The children are born Deaf or become Deaf shortly after birth. Their family members are all hearing, as is the case for most Deaf people. Approximately 75% of hearing parents do not sign with their Deaf children, choosing to communicate via a small set of gestures, speaking, and lipreading. This context leads to the possibility for a child to develop a homesign system. It has been shown that it is the Deaf children who create homesign systems, not their parents, which we will discuss in more detail later in this chapter.

The phenomenon of children developing their own communication system occurs all over the world, including the United States. The primary factors include limited to no exposure to a signed or spoken language, being isolated from other Deaf children/adults, and parental choices with respect to communication with their child. Children of hearing parents frequently create their own gestural system in the absence of linguistic input, i.e., they use homesigns. Many, if not most, Deaf children of hearing parents start out with a self-created gestural system they use for communication with their parents and families, which then is dropped when they enter school, either a school for Deaf children or into a mainstreamed program at a public or private school.

Moreover, some of these Deaf children who have created their own homesign system do not go to school or only go to school for a short time; therefore, they are not exposed to a conventional sign language or to a spoken language, so they grow up using their self-created linguistic system and become adult homesigners.

Young homesigners differ from adult homesigners in some significant ways with respect to their individual homesign systems. It has to be emphasized that all of these homesign systems are created idiosyncratically, with little input from the parents or other members of the family. In researching these homesign systems, we do not expect to see all of the homesign systems contain the same "grammar," just as we know that not all languages have the same grammar. However, homesign systems share some features with each other and even with full languages. This helps to address major questions of linguistics, as we consider what all languages or linguistic systems have in common with respect to their structure, and what governs the variation between these languages and linguistic systems.

7.2.1 Components of a homesign system

First, let's look at the components presented in homesign systems of Deaf children and how they compare to child acquisition of language. Research on homesigners has shown that certain properties of language appear even without input. Different groups of young homesigners show similar properties in their systems, even across cultures as distinct as American and Chinese.

Ten young Deaf children of hearing parents, ranging in age from 1;04 to 4;11 were involved in a large research study. One homesigner, "David," created the most extensive gestural system, having produced the greatest number of utterances in the data collected compared to the other children in the study, so we will focus on his system. David produced in his gestural system evidence of certain properties of language, for example, a lexicon of words he made up, a tendency to use a particular word order, and complex sentences with more than one proposition, among others. We will expand on these three components.

David produced 190 different gestures, but out of these, 81 were used only once in the data. In the remaining 109 gestures, David rarely changed the form of the gesture across different occurrences. This indicates that he is consistent in the use of the signs he created. Furthermore, each gesture token is associated with a particular meaning, providing even more evidence of systematicity. His gestures could also be combined with other gestures to create a new compound gesture, showing productivity. He also had noun–verb pairs, such as JAR and TWIST-OPEN, in which both gestures share the same root handshape and lexical relationship, but they are signed in a way to delineate the two; in particular, the noun is signed once and the verb is repeated twice. This process is similar to that seen in ASL as discussed in Chapter 3, but ASL uses the opposite pattern, i.e., the noun is produced with a repeated motion and the verb is produced with a single motion.

The word order pattern in David's and other homesigners' gestural systems was also studied and a systematic pattern was found. When the action conveyed is *intransitive*, i.e., there is an agent and an action but no other participants, then the gesture for the actor appears before the gesture for the action. For example, a homesigner would sign an intransitive construction with the actor first, such as MOUSE RUN. When the action is *transitive*, i.e., the action has an effect on a patient, then the gesture for the patient occurs before the gesture for the action. For example, if a homesigner signed MOUSE BITE, this would most likely mean that the mouse was bitten by something, meaning the mouse is the *patient*, rather than that the mouse bit something (as it would if it were the actor in a transitive construction). These two sentence types show that homesigners exhibited a preference for the action gesture to be in the utterance-final position. Complex sentences, in which there is more than one proposition in one sentence, were also produced. For instance, David signed CLAP-David-TWIST-BLOW-Mother, meaning that he wants his mother to open the jar and blow a bubble for him to clap.

7.2.2 Cross-cultural comparisons of homesigners

When a group of young homesigners in Taiwan (Republic of China), ages 3;08 to 4;09, were studied in comparison to American homesigners (ages 2;10 to 4;11), there was little difference found between the two groups in terms of syntactic structure used in their homesign systems. Both groups tended to communicate using sentences composed of more than one gesture instead of the single gestures so often favored by the primary caretaker. As in the American group discussed above, the Chinese homesigners indicated a similar preference for word order with the transitive *patient* and the intransitive *actor* in the same, preverbal position. The Chinese homesigners also produced complex sentences in their gestural system.

This is an interesting comparison because the two groups are geographically and culturally far from each other, but yet, they produce very similar gestural systems with respect to their syntax. The researchers did find that the mothers of the Chinese home-signers produced more similar gestures in form and syntax than the American mothers did with their children, which might be due to cultural or paralinguistic considerations. However, there was variability within each group; that is, the individual home-signers had their own sets of gestures that differed from the others for the same type of object or predicate. For this reason, another study examined the morphological form in the gestural systems of these two groups, asking whether the group-internal differences could be attributed to cultural influences or parental input.

Three types of shared gestures between the caregivers and the young homesigners were observed in communication between the dyads: a "hold-up" gesture in which the person holds up an object and points to it; conventional gestures that are commonly used between hearing people such as "give" (palm-up and out-stretched), "sleep" (palm on side of face and head tilted), "nod-ding yes" (head nods up and down), and "don't know" (palms turning and facing up); and iconic gestures in which the hands describe a particular action or shape of an object. In this study, the iconic gestures were examined because this is where the most morphological variation occurs. There are multiple ways to de-scribe actions and objects by looking at their handshapes and movement (see Chapter 2 for more discussion on these terms). The children use handshapes to represent objects, to show the form used when handling objects, or to trace the movement of an object. For example, a hat was represented in two ways by one of the homesigners: using the handshape of a fist ✊ as in pulling the hat down on your head, or with the handshape of a flat hand ✋ showing the shape of the bill of the hat. Another child used the 𝒞 handshape to represent a type of object being handled such as a horn or the shape of a cowboy's bowed legs while on a horse.

In the study, all of the children and the mothers used iconic gestures, with the mothers using them less often than the children. The Chinese mothers used almost as many different forms of handshapes and motions as their children but the American mothers used significantly less than either their children or the Chinese mothers. Comparing between the American and Chinese homesigners, it was found that each group exhibited similarity in handshapes and motions used for particular objects, e.g., ✆ for grasping or a round object. Interestingly enough, there were some handshapes used in a particular way by the American homesigners but not by the Chinese homesigners. A ♟ handshape was used to illustrate something in contact with a large surface or a series of small surfaces by the American homesigners, but the Chinese homesigners only used this handshape for something in contact with a large surface. To some degree, there were many similarities between the two groups in the handshapes and motions chosen for objects and movement, but there were still some idiosyncratic choices reserved by individual homesigners, such as using the index finger to represent a vehicle, or using the ♟ handshape to show two skinny objects, which was observed with all but one of the homesigners.

How much of the gestural variation between homesigners came from the mother's input to their child? In the same study, the mothers' use of handshapes and motions were compared to their child's use of the same. Less than half of what the mothers used to describe/name an object or its movement was the same for their child. In other words, the mother and the child did not have the same gestural system as would be expected if the mother's input was the source for the child's gestural system. Another example of this is illustrated in a different study in which three young American homesigners (who did not know each other) all incorporated the gesture for WAIT-A-MINUTE into their system but used it to signify the "immediate future" as in "I'm going to do this next," rather than an instruction to stop. However, none of their mothers used the gesture in the same way their child did, but instead they used its conventional meaning, i.e., "stop." The parents do not use the same gestures in the same way as the children do. That is, the children's linguistic system was not typically adopted and used by the parents in the same manner. The parents typically appropriated indexical gestures and used gestures that accompanied their speech but did not apply the same conventions to the gestures that their children did.

Another surprising finding is that the child's gestural system was far more likely to overlap that of another homesigner than their own mother, regardless of which culture they were from. So, not only did the study not find many within-group differences but also there were no significant differences in the use of gestures between the two cultural groups of young homesigners. What does this tell us? It tells us that humans can and will utilize innate mechanisms to create a linguistic system for communication.

7.3 Adult homesigners

As mentioned earlier, most young homesigners eventually go on to learn either the spoken language or signed language predominantly used in their country, either at a school with mostly hearing children or at a school for the Deaf. However, there are deaf adults who were never exposed to a language, or first experienced exposure to a given language (either signed or spoken) at a very late age, in their 40s and 50s. Typically, we find adult homesigners living in remote, rural regions of countries that have few or no services for the Deaf. As mentioned earlier in this chapter, homesign systems have been found all over the world, even in economically developed countries, albeit usually in areas that are geographically isolated. For example, there are many adult homesigners who live in remote areas of the Appalachian Mountains in the United States. In Brazil, homesigners live in "favelas," crowded, low-income communities developed among the hills that are almost impossible to navigate via car. The linguistic system that they created as young homesigners becomes refined as they grow into adulthood using it for communication with everyone. That is, as children, they typically use their self-generated system to communicate primarily with parents and family. Adult homesigners use their gestural system to communicate with peers, parents, family, and people they meet in their community.

Both young and adult homesigners produce a lexicon in which the homesigner develops a mental list of gestures consistently used for a particular item or action. Not only that, the gestures used by their primary caretaker often differ from those of the homesigner.

A group of researchers studied the lexicons developed individually by seven homesigners, ranging in age from 11 to 33 years, and studied whether items in that lexicon are shared with their communication partners, i.e., their relatives or friends. The researchers wanted to know if both the homesigner and his or her communication partner consistently use the same form for the same object. The researchers showed the participants pictures of everyday objects such as an orange, a cow, or a potato, and asked them to produce a gesture for the object. Significant variability in the responses from the homesigner and their communication partner was observed; i.e., they did not share the same gesture for the designated object. Moreover, each homesigner was more consistent in their designation for the items than their own communication partner, and the homesigners also had more differentiated gestures than their communication partners. What this means is that they developed a more fine-grained lexicon whereas their communication partners would employ the same gesture for different items.

Recent studies suggest that differences also exist between the linguistic systems of young homesigners and adult homesigners with respect to complexity and word order. Studies with Nicaraguan and Brazilian homesigners have produced evidence of several sophisticated linguistic components, including the presence of a subject as a grammatical category differentiated from topic, structural hierarchy, and noun–noun compounding. We will now discuss these aspects in more depth.

When an adult homesigner's system is studied, the question arises as to whether their system distinguishes a particular noun phrase functioning as a subject, i.e., a distinct grammatical category that all mature, formal languages have. An alternative possibility is that the noun phrases in question function as topics, which on some views would require positing less grammatical complexity.

In one study, three adult homesigners, ages 15, 19, and 24 at the time of the most recent analyses, were tested according to their ability to distinguish between two grammatical categories – the subject and the topic in their own homesign system. The researchers investigated the grammatical category subject using elicited production tasks in which the participant signs a description of events depicted in a series of pictures. Each of the homesigners consistently used the same word order to indicate the subject of the utterance, regardless of its semantic role as agent, patient, or experiencer. The word order was not always the same across the homesigners but for each homesigner, in their own system, the word order was consistent. In another experiment, they were also able to distinguish between the subject and the topic in their productions. The results of these experiments indicate that these two grammatical categories are explicitly distinguished in the homesign systems, despite the homesigners' having had little or no exposure to a source language with these categories.

More evidence of a relatively high level of complexity has been observed in a study with Brazilian adult homesigners, who show evidence of noun–noun compounding, embedded clauses, and clauses with structure dependency. Compounding in ASL was introduced in Chapter 3. Here we focus on recursive noun–noun compounding, which requires the ability to combine nouns multiple times. In English, examples such as "Christmas program book" or "cat lady house" illustrate recursive noun–noun compounding. In one study, Brazilian adult homesigners created noun–noun compounds such as BEAR FRAME PHOTO "bear picture frame." They also created sentences with more than one proposition, as illustrated in (1a, b), and different types of phrases, as in (1c). In (1a) and (1b), the constructions have a sentence within a larger sentence, i.e., embedding. In (1c), there is a locative phrase, a noun phrase, and a verb phrase. One homesigner produced examples (1a) and (1b); another produced example (1c).

1 a PT-(ME) THINK BABY PT-(ME) SMALL
      "I think I was a small baby."

   b REMEMBER PATH LOC AROUND-THERE SLEEP
      AROUND-THERE MANY MEOW
      "I remember there were many cats sleeping around this
      path over there."

   c PT-(OUT-THERE), HOUSE-ROOF, PLANE-FLY-OVER
      over-there, house, plane fly over
      "The plane flew over the house."

The Brazilian homesigners also exhibit further evidence of linguistic structure via a relation called *structure dependency*. Structure dependency is when one grammatical category is dependent on the appearance of another, i.e., the word order is hierarchically structured at an abstract level, not dependent on a string of words or sequential order. According to the hypothesis that languages systematically display structure dependency, words must be grouped together to create phrases according to a consistent pattern or rule. For instance, in English, we cannot say *The boy kicked the ball small is* or *The boy kicked small the ball*. The adjective "small" has to occur immediately before the noun "ball." It's not enough to say it has to occur before the noun as we see in the second example. Homesigners show structure dependency by consistently producing adjectives or modifiers with the noun they modify; i.e., we do not see instances where a modifier occurs in a position away from the noun that it modifies, such as *"MAN HUG BIG," with the intended meaning "the big man hugs."

Some examples produced by three Brazilian homesigners of nouns and their modifiers are presented in (2) below. One thing to note is that the ordering allows the modifier to be either before or after the noun, but the noun and its modifier are not separated. One homesigner produced (2a) and (2b). The other two homesigners in the study produced (2c) and (2d) respectively.

2   a   [[SMALL BORN-BABY] GOOD
         "(A) small newly birthed baby is good."

    b   [[BAG PT(bag)] PUT-IN PT]
          bag   that   put-in you

         "You can put (the stuff) in the bag."

    c   [[MAN BIG] HUG]]
         "(The) big man hugged (the bear)."

    d   [PT [SMALL BABY]] GROW-UP], PT
         "That small baby grew up."

Another interesting observation is that studies with Brazilian and Nicaraguan adult homesigners show that their multi-gesture utterances do not exhibit the pattern exhibited by the young homesigners discussed earlier in this chapter. These homesigners instead present a strong preference for subject–verb ordering, with either transitive or intransitive verbs.

In sum, studies of adult homesigners indicate that their systems show a greater complexity, including compounding, consistent marking of grammatical roles, and same-category recursion not seen in young homesigners, perhaps as a result of maturity or increased self-generated input from interacting with the environment and more conversation partners. From the studies summarized above and others, we can see that homesigners develop a linguistic system that is language-like, even if such systems still lack certain features found in established, mature languages. We have presented evidence that homesign systems are not based primarily on input provided by gestures produced by parents and other conversation partners. The conversation partners' gestures are more limited and less structured than those of the homesigners. Therefore, the homesigners are the source of the innovation of the linguistic system rather than the mothers or family members who are their communication partners. Homesigners experience no access to syntactic phenomena in either a spoken or signed language. Homesigners clearly experience greatly impoverished input, and yet, they produce evidence of grammatical phenomena in their linguistic system. This result provides a strong argument for some form of innate linguistic knowledge despite "poverty of the stimulus."

7.4 Homesigners' acquisition of a conventional signed language

As mentioned earlier, oftentimes a homesigner will learn a conventional community signed language later, upon meeting other Deaf children at school or others in the community. One might wonder how well they acquire this signed language. Do they acquire it as a first language or a second language? As we have seen in Chapter 5, Deaf people who learn a given signed language as their first language from birth compare similarly to typically developing hearing children acquiring their spoken language as a first language. The milestones are similar, and they gain higher levels of proficiency and processing than those who acquire the same language as late learners.

A few studies have observed the acquisition of a signed language by Deaf homesigners. David, who was prolific in his creation of gestures in his linguistic system as a young homesigner, later learned ASL and was tested on his ability to produce and distinguish classifier verbs of motion in ASL (see Chapter 3) two times – once when he was nine and half years old with little exposure to ASL at that time, and later when he was 23 years old, having learned ASL by then.

In the first study, his ability to produce ASL-like morphemes with respect to location and motion was no different from native signers. He could distinguish between different types of movement for different objects in motion. However, the handshapes he used to represent the objects in motion were significantly different from those used in ASL by native signers. For instance, he used the same handshape to represent anything cylindrical, making flat round objects indistinguishable from round cylindrical objects, and he used the 👍 handshape instead of the 🖐 handshape used for vehicles in ASL.

Later, in the second study with the same test, David's acquisition of ASL exhibited similar patterns to those who learned ASL as a late first language. He did well when the handshape morphemes in ASL overlapped with those from his homesign system. If there was a new handshape in typical ASL that he had never used, or for which he had used a different one in his homesign system, he did not do as well in producing the correct ASL handshape.

It can be concluded that even though learning a language and self-creating a language utilizes similar innate mechanisms, if one learns a source language later in life, their acquisition will not be the equivalent to either native signers (L1 learners) or L2 signers. In some ways, the homesign system provides a foundation for learning a conventional sign language later, but not in the same way a first language would for L2 learners. So, when a homesigner learns ASL later, they are considered to be a late learner of ASL rather than an L2 learner (unless they have had enough exposure to English for it to serve as a L1). They do well in creating their own self-generated linguistic system with many language-like components, but not as well in processing and grammaticalization of a full system.

7.5 Conclusion

There continues to be more research on homesign systems because they provide a fascinating window into language creation in a way that we could not otherwise duplicate in research. Homesigners, young and adult, rely on a gestural system to communicate with the world outside, but as shown above, this is in the face of severely impoverished input. Their caregivers or primary communication partners do not share the system created by the homesigner, instead relying on their own much smaller constellation of gestures. In other words, homesigners utilize their system to express their thoughts, but do not have the benefit of receptive information, which is quite different from children (Deaf and hearing) acquiring a target language as a first language who have both expressive and receptive modes utilized at a high rate. Homesigners have been shown to have a lower range of topics, a more limited lexicon, and a lower rate of gesturing than comparable Deaf signing or hearing speaking children. Even though they self-generate a linguistic system without input from a source language and show many language-like components that are capable of conveying their thoughts, feelings, and ideas, the system is primarily for their expressive use. They are still very much linguistically and socially isolated. The issue of language deprivation is very real for Deaf children, especially for homesigners who experience a double degree of language poverty with no or little exposure to either signed or spoken language. Language is a right that all children should have, with full accessibility of both expressive and receptive modes.

Discussion questions

1   How are homesign systems similar to natural languages? How are they different?

2   How do we know that homesign systems are invented by children and not based on the input they receive from their caregivers?
3   Why do you think children invent a homesign system?
4   What does the fact that homesign systems exist tell us about how humans naturally acquire a language? In what ways do you think self-generation of a homesign system is different from acquiring a source language?

Further reading

Coppola, M., & Newport, E. L. (2005). Grammatical subjects in home sign: abstract linguistic structure in adult primary gesture systems without linguistic input. *Proceedings of the National Academy of Sciences of the United States of America, 102*(52), 19249–19253.
This paper describes the study discussed in this chapter about how adult homesigners have a grammatical category of subject.

Goldin-Meadow, S. (2003). *The Resilience of language: what gesture creation in deaf children can tell us about how all children learn language.* New York, NY: Psychology Press.
This book is a classic in homesign research, as Dr. Goldin-Meadow was the first to study young homesigners.

Morford, J. P. (1996). Insights to language from the study of gesture: a review of research on the gestural communication of non-signing deaf people. *Language and Communication, 16*(2), 165–172.
A nice overview of all the research on homesign systems and homesigners.

Richie, R., Yang, C., & Coppola, M. (2014). Modeling the emergence of lexicons in homesign systems. *Topics in Cognitive Science, 6*(1), 183–195.
A fascinating study of how homesigners developed a lexicon for their system.

Bibliography

Coppola, M. (2002). *The emergence of grammatical categories in home sign: evidence from family-based gesture systems in Nicaragua* (Dissertation). University of Rochester, Rochester, NY.

Goldin-Meadow, S. (2003a). The resilience of language. In B. Beachley, A. Brown, & F. Conlin (Eds.), *Proceedings of the 27th Annual Boston University Conference on Language Development* (Vol. 27, pp. 1–25). Somerville, MA: Cascadilla Press.

Goldin-Meadow, S. (2005). What language creation in the manual modality tells us about the foundations of language. *Linguistic Review, 22*, 199–225.

Goldin-Meadow, S., & Mylander, C. (2007). Spontaneous sign systems created by deaf children in two cultures. *Cognitive Psychology, 55*(2), 87–135.

Goldin-Meadow, S., Mylander, C., & Franklin, A. (2007). How children make language out of gesture: morphological structure in gesture systems developed by American and Chinese deaf children. *Cognitive Psychology, 55*, 87–135.

Morford, J. P., & Hänel-Faulhaber, B. (2011). Homesigners as late learners: Connecting the dots from delayed acquisition in childhood to sign language processing in adulthood. *Language and Linguistics Compass, 5*(8), 525–537.

Morford, J. P., & Kegl, J. (2000). Gestural precursors to linguistic constructs: how input shapes the form of language. In D. McNeill (Ed.), *Language and gesture* (pp. 358–387). Cambridge, England: Cambridge University Press.

Morford, J. P., Singleton, J. L., & Goldin-Meadow, S. (1995). The genesis of language: how much time is needed to generate arbitrary symbols in a sign system? In K. Emmorey & J. Reilly (Eds.), *Language, gesture, and space* (pp. 313–332). Hillsdale, NJ: Lawrence Erlbaum Associates.

Richie, R., Fanghella, J., & Coppola, M. (2012). Emergence of lexicons in family-based homesign systems in Nicaragua. In Geer, L. C. (Ed.), *Proceedings from the 13th Meeting of the Texas Linguistics Society* (pp. 55–67). Austin, TX: University of Texas.

Senghas, A. (2003). Intergenerational influence and ontogenetic development in the emergence of spatial grammar in Nicaraguan Sign Language. *Cognitive Development, 18*, 511–531.

Senghas, A., & Coppola, M. (2001). Children creating language: how Nicaraguan Sign Language acquired a spatial grammar. *Psychological Science, 12*(4), 323–328.

Singleton, J. L., Morford, J. P., & Goldin-Meadow, S. (1993). Once is not enough: standards of well-formedness in manual communication created over three different timespans. *Language, 69*, 683–715.

Supalla, T., & Newport, E. L. (1978). How many seats in a chair? The derivation of nouns and verbs in American Sign Language. In P. Siple (Ed.), *Understanding Language through Sign Language Research* (pp. 91–132). New York, NY: Academic Press.

Wood, S., & Morford, J. P. (2016). Psycholinguistics: gestures & home signs. In G. Gertz & P. Bouldreault (Eds.), *The SAGE deaf studies encyclopedia*. Los Angeles, CA: SAGE Publications.

Chapter 8

Variation

This chapter begins a section of the book on sociolinguistics. Every linguistic community has its own set of practices; some may be shared among several communities, and others may be unique to one particular community. Culture also influences how a language is practiced in a particular context with people at a given time. For these reasons, there is a need to have a social component in a linguistic theory that accounts for sociocultural factors related to similarities and differences between language varieties, which will be discussed in this chapter. In the next two chapters, we will discuss language attitudes based on the societal views of language, and language policy and planning related to language practices, language ideology, and language maintenance.

8.1 Sociocultural components in linguistic theories

Certain linguistic patterns appear to be used and structured differently in sign and spoken languages due to the different communication modalities; for example, a signer articulates with multiple body parts including hands, torso, head, and face to produce signed expressions and a speaker articulates with different parts of the mouth, vocal folds, and lungs to produce spoken expressions. As the preceding chapters have shown, we can use analytical tools to describe linguistic features and patterns, and there are linguistic theories to explain why languages are structured and function in certain ways, whether signed or spoken. However, linguistic theories alone cannot account for variation that exists within languages; for example, why the English words "potato," "aunt," and "water" are each pronounced differently by different people, and why we have more than ten different signs for BIRTHDAY in American Sign Language (ASL). Sociocultural and historical practices are where we need to look to explain variation of this type.

8.2 Conditions affecting language use and variation

Factors such as cultural diversity, political conditions, historical influences, and geographic regions explain the social and geographic boundaries of the world's languages, signed and spoken. Some language communities can coexist comfortably with each other, but for others, their coexistence can be uncomfortable or even contentious. As in the cases of social differences between communities, languages are often tied to different domains such that a language or dialect may be acceptable in certain domains but not in others. Domains are the abstract representations of time, setting, and relationships combined in a certain way that define expectations and values for linguistic and communication behaviors including language use. Typical domains for language use include family, friendship, employment, education, religion, and neighborhood. People change their linguistic behaviors in different domains depending on when it is, where they are, and who they are with. As one hypothetical example, suppose a group of Mexican American students behave in a certain way with their teacher in a classroom and use standard English as expected at school; when the school lets out, the students who are also neighbors use Spanglish (a mixture of Spanish and English) on the way home. At home, the parents of one of the students are Mexican immigrants and they prefer to speak Spanish in this domain. It just so happens that the family are close with their Deaf relatives who use Mexican Sign Language (LSM) so when the relatives visit, everyone uses LSM out of respect for the guests. So far, we have identified three different domains for four different language varieties: standard English at school, Spanglish with school friends, and Spanish and LSM at home.

The frequency and specificity of language use within certain domains is not random; it is related to social differences that function as linguistic boundaries due to institutional and social pressures. Every culture has some form of social stratification that categorizes social differences in a hierarchal manner from superior to inferior based on status, power and prestige. Since language is a social tool, it can function as an indicator of one's status, identity, and character. Within formal domains such as education, employment, and legal settings, people feel compelled to use a standard language or dialect within the area where social hierarchy is emphasized or noticeable. Outside of formal domains, they use a social language where there is less emphasis on social hierarchy, but social differences can still be a defining factor in linguistic boundaries (see Chapter 9 for further discussion on social stratification and its effect on linguistic prestige). The relationship between domains and social stratification creates a *diglossic* function for language varieties.

Diglossia is a situation where language varieties including languages and dialects are used under different conditions within the same community, and such varieties are differentiated by formality and prestige. Formal varieties are called "high" varieties and informal varieties are called "low" varieties. People usually acquire high varieties through socialization in formal domains and rarely at home with family and friends, whereas low varieties are acquired in informal settings. Varieties are compartmentalized according to the social domains wherever their use is appropriate. Going back to the example of the Mexican American students, standard English is commonly accepted as a high variety, and the other varieties used by these students are considered low varieties. Suppose the family of the student whose parents are immigrants returns to Mexico City due to job relocation; then the diglossic situation is different. In this context, Spanish is now the high variety at school and work. Spanglish is generally discouraged in Mexico so the student only uses it when communicating with American friends online. English is a bit tricky since it is predominantly used as a lingua franca around the world, but in this case, Spanish is the dominant language. If English is used, it is for specific domains such as when meeting with English speakers or giving a presentation at an international conference; but generally in Mexico Spanish is to be expected. Interestingly, LSM is not highly regarded in the United States or in Mexico so it is a low variety either way, even though LSM is native to Mexico. This presents a question about sign languages: are they highly regarded anywhere? (See Chapter 9 on language attitudes).

8.2.1 Factors in the formation and maintenance of sign languages

Sign language communities can be subjected to similar institutional and social conditions as those that influence language practices of the spoken-language communities. Among the world's languages, over 130 sign languages have been counted, but how sign languages are counted and categorized as separate languages or dialects of one language is not always clear or consistent. Nevertheless, the count of sign languages is reliably well over 100. In the history of humanity, the earliest known reference to the use of a sign language can be found in the philosophy book of Plato, *Cratylus*, which is a dialogue about language. One quote made by Socrates is as follows:

> If we hadn't a voice or a tongue, and wanted to express things to one another, wouldn't we try to make signs by moving our hands, head, and the rest of our body, just as dumb people do at present?

By "dumb," Socrates refers to people who couldn't speak and hear (see discussion of language ideology in Chapter 10). This is one of the earliest written records about the use of signs, but it doesn't mean that no signed communication systems had existed before the 5th century BC. Humans are driven to communicate with each other by any means, and disability including deafness has been part of the whole history of humanity, so it is entirely possible that there were instances of sign languages between Deaf people prior to that time. However, the modern history of stable signing communities is fairly recent with the development of public education for deaf children.

Education is a common factor in the maintenance and transmission of sign languages. Starting in the 1770s when the world's first public institution for deaf students was established in Paris,

France, the school became an educational model with sign language as a medium of instruction for those involved in deaf education. In this case, because the first school was in France, it was French Sign Language (LSF, Langue des Signes Française) that was used. This model inspired the establishment of educational institutions as government-funded residential schools with specialized educational services for deaf children. What drove this deaf education movement was religion, a common motivation in establishing educational institutions, with sign languages as an accessible means of communication so the educators could teach deaf students religious subjects. During the 18th and 19th centuries, it was typical for religious professionals such as nuns and priests to work as educators and administrators at deaf schools. The enrollment age of deaf children could be as young as toddler or much later – the modern early hearing detection and intervention technology did not exist at that time, so deafness was usually identified much later. The majority of deaf children were born to hearing families who did not sign, which severely limited their language input, unless families used home signs with them (see Chapter 7 on homesign). Once families knew about these schools, they would send their children away to them if possible. A sudden family separation was a traumatic event for deaf children, especially if their parents could not explain to them why they could not stay at home with their family anymore given limited communication. After a while, once the newcomers were able to connect linguistically with their peers and the adults at the school, the signing of their cohorts and educators would bring comfort to them. Such institutions became the regular basis for deaf children to acquire sign language and the foundation of modern signing communities, including Australian Sign Language (Auslan), Lingua Brasileira de Sinais (Libras), British Sign Language (BSL), LSF, ASL, and Hong Kong Sign Language (HKSL).

However, not all Deaf people in the world acquire a sign language at school. There are sign languages that were created within communities where there are a significant number of members who are deaf due to genetics or acquired disability. Those communities are sign language microcommunities that include indigenous, rural, or village sign languages. The reason for the high incidence of deafness in the microcommunities compared to that observed in sign language macrocommunities is often related to a high number of intermarriages with close family members. Sign language researchers have come across communities that have generations of people with different hearing abilities using the indigenous sign languages, for example, in Alipur, India; Chican, Mexico; Bedouin Arab communities in Israel; Adamorabe, Ghana; and so on. Unfortunately, the communities are vulnerable to economic and socio-political pressures that affect their local economic and sociocultural power and they may be especially vulnerable to pressures relating to educational, medical, and technological advances in the intervention of deafness.

These same pressures are also a constant threat to stable signing communities via shifts in deaf education, medical intervention, and technological advances. In the 19th century, speech as the sole instructional method for deaf children gained popularity in Germany and nearby countries, and this approach, also known as oralism, became a threat to the signing method. The threat became a reality in 1880 at the International Congress on Education of the Deaf in Milan, Italy, where the majority of educators voted to discontinue sign language as an instructional method, despite the passionate objection from the minority who supported the signing method. Most attendees viewed sign language as a hindrance to the integration of deaf children with the society where speech was the norm. It can be argued that their view was shaped by the national and international contexts, including the interplay of nationalist sentiments, competing economic powers, and technological innovations. With the oral method viewed as a practical innovative model that could easily be taught, it edged out the signing method for a few reasons: it was time-consuming for educators to learn a sign language; the instruction of sign language was expensive to maintain; and the participants believed that the signing method had outlived its usefulness in the age of science that demanded efficiency. In spite of the ban on the use of the sign language method, sign languages were still used by deaf children at their schools mainly because of their accessibility.

Sign languages survived in spite of physical punishments and emotional traumas that deaf children had to endure at the hand of educators and administrators who were committed to the speech-only ideology at all cost. Unfortunately, the speech-only ideology still exists today with the promotion of listening and speaking or audio-verbal therapy and hearing intervention services. Such promotion is coupled with the misguided notion that sign language could impair language development in deaf children and therefore should be avoided. Through legal and advocacy support, Deaf communities are responding to the ideological threat by raising awareness about the nature of sign languages and Deaf culture and promoting educational materials and training (see further discussion on language ideology and language policy and planning in Chapter 10). The contention within the educational, political, and social domains shapes how sign languages have come to exist the way they are and how they are related historically and culturally.

8.2.2 Families of sign languages in historical, linguistic, and social contexts

Like spoken languages, sign languages can be grouped into language families which are based on similarity of linguistic features and structure as well as shared historical and cultural origins. However, the history of individual sign languages may not follow the same history as spoken languages in their respective nations. For example, the presence of English in the United States is the result of British colonization before the American Revolution in 1775, but ASL has a different history. As noted in Chapter 1, when the American School for the Deaf (ASD) was founded in Hartford, Connecticut in 1817, a Deaf community was formed. The various sign systems used by these community members and the French Sign Language (LSF) used by Laurent Clerc, the school's Deaf co-founder and teacher, merged into ASL. The import of LSF was more of a historical accident because of the chance meeting between Clerc and Reverend Thomas Hopkins Gallaudet. Gallaudet, who was also the hearing cofounder of the ASD, went to England first for the purpose of learning how to educate deaf children. He visited the Braidwood family, who taught deaf children through the oral method. The family was not willing to share their teaching method with Gallaudet. It was by chance that Gallaudet was in a public square where he saw a teaching demonstration by the director of the National Institute for Deaf

Children of Paris, Abbé Sicard, and the Deaf educators Clerc and Jean Massieu. Gallaudet was not able to learn the signing method in a short time so he convinced Clerc to move to America to found the deaf school there. This explains why BSL and ASL are not related despite the history of English imperialism and migration in America.

There is a considerable influence from French Sign Language on ASL based on this history. The influence can be seen in the high percentage of cognates, which are signs that have a high degree of similarity across the languages, and in shared grammatical structures. Based on this fact, LSF and ASL are relatively more mutually intelligible than ASL and BSL, even though the latter share a history of colonization and the spoken language used in the surrounding hearing community. As it goes for any language, when a sign language is imported from another country, eventually it will deviate from its parent sign language. The separation of the languages will grow when the geographical distance functions as a barrier between the two languages, and the parent community's social practices give way to new and modified forms in the child language. Since ASL is a descendant of the older form of LSF, it is classified in the same language family as the modern form of LSF, which includes sign languages in Italy, Denmark, Ireland, and Mexico, for example.

Figure 8.1 shows how a selected sample of sign languages developed as LSF was exported through the education of deaf students with a sign language as the accepted medium of instruction. LSF was imported to America through the founding of the ASD in 1817, and it was combined with the other existing sign systems brought in by deaf children. It eventually gave birth to ASL, which spread throughout the country through the founding of other deaf schools (see Figure 8.2 in Section 8.3).

In the 1950s, Andrew Foster was the first black Deaf college graduate from Gallaudet University, the world's first postsecondary institution for deaf students in Washington, DC. Foster continued with his advanced education and completed two master's degrees from Eastern Michigan University and Seattle Pacific Christian College. As a Christian missionary, he felt a calling to establish the first deaf school in the entire African continent in Ghana and brought his ASL variety as the medium of instruction.

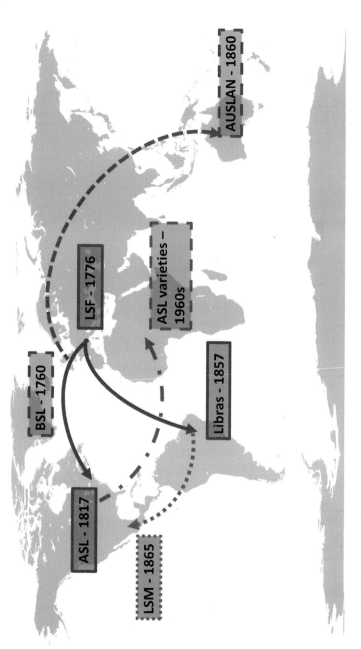

Figure 8.1 The spread of sign languages.

Before his death in 1987, he had founded 31 deaf schools in 13 African countries. Foster is still revered as the father of deaf education in Africa.

In Brazil, LSF was also imported with the founding of the first government-supported school by a Deaf teacher from Paris, Padre Eduarado Huet, in 1857. Huet eventually moved on to Mexico City and founded another first government-supported school, the Escuela San Juan Letran, in 1865.

Many additional examples are not illustrated in Figure 8.1. It could be estimated that over 20 sign language descendants are historically and structurally related to LSF, which was the language of the model school for the world. Even though BSL is not structurally related to ASL, it does have its own language family that includes Australian Sign Language (Auslan) and New Zealand Sign Language (NZSL) as its descendants. Education and geography are two factors that help to explain the linguistic and cultural relationships between sign languages in the world, but there are other factors that also must be identified to explain the differences between sign languages, especially their own dialects.

8.3 Variation within sign languages

In any language, dialects are formed based on external conditions (e.g., social and geographic factors) as well as internal language conditions (e.g., rule extension, analogy, grammaticalization, phonological processes, and word formation processes) that usually co-occur with the external conditions. In the linguistic sense, dialects are structurally related varieties that differ by phonological, lexical, morphological, syntactic, and discourse features. Such varieties exhibit systematic rule-based differences, irrespective of whether they are accepted or not in the society. From a popular perspective, dialects are some forms of language that are considered nonstandard with stigmatized linguistic features, which are only good for social purposes, not for professional or academic purposes. According to the popular perspective, standard language varieties are excluded from the category of dialects because they are perceived to be free of stigmatized linguistic features, but that is not the viewpoint of linguistics, which considers the standard variety as a dialect as well. Standard dialects are aspired to because they contain features that are associated with social, economic, and educational advantages. Because they are modeled as standard, the socially favored features are perceived to be unmarked. The features that are socially disfavored are marked based on their association with marginalized or stigmatized communities (see Chapter 9 on the notion of standard and prestige).

8.3.1 Geographical factors in variation

Factors that define the differences and similarities between dialects include geographic isolation, settlement patterns, migration, and language contact. Geographic isolation consists of natural barriers (e.g., rivers, mountains, and deserts) or artificial barriers (e.g. train tracks, highways, and walls) that physically separate language communities from one another and reduce the chance of language contact between communities. When the communities have a reduced chance of face to face communication on a personal level with one another, this increases the chance of divergence in linguistic forms where changes occur in one community but do not occur in the others. Over time, such changes will build up until the differences between dialects will be obvious. Such a progression explains the number of North American dialects of English that are based on geographical origins: Northeast American English, Southern American English, Pacific Northwest dialect, Appalachian English, New York City English, and Pittsburghese (which is a dialect used in Pittsburgh). The geographical regions do not have to be necessarily large; geographically based dialectal differences can be found within a state, county, and even neighborhood, depending on how limited the contact is between the communities. Dialects can also be traced alongside the migration routes taken by the earliest inhabitants from their original settlements; the trace of migration routes follows natural geographic barriers such as mountains, rivers, and lakes.

As can be seen in Figure 8.2, the ASL variety created in Hartford, Connecticut, was eventually spread throughout the country via the establishment of deaf schools. With the geographical isolation of deaf schools, sign variants emerged in different regions through creativity and interaction between signing peers at the deaf schools

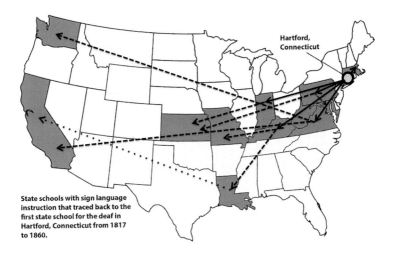

Hartford, Connecticut

State schools with sign language instruction that traced back to the first state school for the deaf in Hartford, Connecticut from 1817 to 1860.

Figure 8.2 The spread of ASL in the United States.

and perhaps contact with indigenous and mainstream communities with existing or innovative forms.

Lexical and phonological variation is one distinct feature that is easily perceptible. The well-known example of the ASL sign for "birthday" illustrates this point. In Figure 8.3a, one version of this sign is shown: the signer touches the chin with the open-8 handshape and then moves the hand down to touch the chest. However, there are other variants for BIRTHDAY (see Figure 8.3) with iconic or semantic meanings related to being born, blowing out candles, tugging on one's ear, wishing happiness, and singing. Those variants are usually geographically bound. The first BIRTHDAY sign in Figure 8.3a is a recognizable form in ASL, which is standardized through education including specialized education programs for deaf students and sign language interpreting programs, but the other variants are still actively used in regional communities.

Variation is not limited to lexical and phonological variation; it can include morphology, syntax, discourse, and style. People are aware of linguistic differences between language varieties, but how they perceive the differences depends on their social

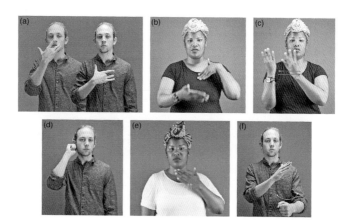

Figure 8.3 Variants of the ASL sign, BIRTHDAY: (a) BIRTHDAY, standard variant; (b) BIRTHDAY-BORN; (c) BIRTHDAY-CANDLES; (d) BIRTHDAY-EAR; (e) BIRTHDAY-HAPPY; and (f) BIRTHDAY-SING. Images: ASL Signbank, 2018.

bias. Dialects with stigmatized features are often associated with groups of people who are in an unfavorable social status with respect to geography, race, ethnicity, class, religion, and generation (see Chapter 9 for further discussion on African American English and Black ASL). For example, Black ASL is an ASL dialect used by black Deaf Southerners. Black ASL was formed during the segregation era when southern and border states mandated racial separation in every area, including schools.

Racial separation is often associated with these geographical factors and can lead to dialects that are associated with particular racial groups (see Figure 8.4). Black deaf children were physically isolated in every sense from white deaf children after the end of the Civil War until the end of state-sanctioned racial segregation. Some states had separate schools for black and white students that were a few hundred miles apart. In North Carolina, for example, the white deaf school in Morganton was about 200 miles from the black deaf school in Raleigh. Some states had schools in the same town; for example, in Talladega, Alabama, the black deaf school was only 15 minutes away from the white deaf school, but not everyone in town was aware of the

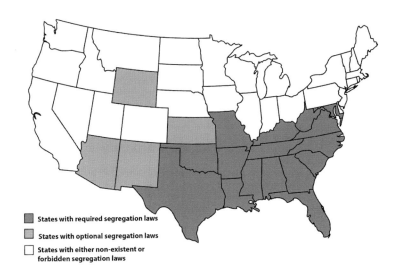

Figure 8.4 Segregation in the southern US states marked in dark gray.

existence of both deaf schools. This shows how strong the force of the racial barrier was. A few schools had a department on the same campus that was designed for black deaf children to be educated in a separate setting from white deaf children, like Kendall Elementary School on the campus of Gallaudet College (later renamed Gallaudet University) in Washington, DC (see Table 8.1).

During the segregation period, black deaf children at the time had virtually no contact with white deaf children. As a result, Black ASL was qualitatively different from the signing of white deaf students and their school staff (see the online material on Black ASL). Sometime after the end of racial segregation in education, black deaf students were admitted to schools for white deaf children, but they felt marked and targeted by their use of Black ASL. They coped by code-switching or adopting the mainstream ASL. As of late, Black ASL is not as stigmatized due to massive linguistic changes as the result of federally mandated racial integration and educational mainstreaming of disabled students.

Table 8.1 Black and white deaf schools: founding and desegregation

State	White school established	Black school/department established	Desegregation	Years between establishment of black and white schools	Years between establishment of black schools and desegregation
DC, KDES	1857	1857 (dept.)	1958	0	101
North Carolina	1845	1868–1869	1967	24	98
Maryland	1868	1872	1956	4	84
Tennessee	1845	1881 (dept.)	1965	36	84
Georgia	1846	1882	1965	36	83
Mississippi	1854	1882 (dept.)	1965	28	83
South Carolina	1849	1883 (dept.)	1966	34	83
Kentucky	1823	1884 (dept.)	1954–1960	61	70
Florida	1885	1885	1965	0	80
Texas	1857	1887	1965	30	78
Arkansas	1850/1867	1887	1967	37	80
Alabama	1858	1892	1968	34	76
Missouri	1861	1888 (dept.)	1954	37	66
Kansas	1861	1888 (dept.)	1954	27	66
Virginia	1839	1909	1965 (2 schools)	70	56
Oklahoma	1898	1909, dept.	1962	11	53
Louisiana	1852	1938	1978	86	40
West Virginia	1870	1926	1956	56	30

Note: Adapted from American Annals of the Deaf (1951 January) McCaskill, Lucas, Bayley, and Hill (2011).

8.3.2 Social factors in variation

Racial separation is counted among the social constraints that define the differences between dialects. Others include social class, caste, age, gender, ethnicity, religion, political factions, and more. Any social identity that is meaningful and powerful enough to set a group apart from another group can be a defining factor in the formation and maintenance of dialects. The study of social factors has evolved in three different waves depending on the innovative research methods and approaches used at each time.

The first wave of sociolinguistic analysis started with William Labov's quantitative research method. In this approach, different speech forms were typically counted and arranged in table form for numerical analysis. Labov's classic sociolinguistic study in 1966 concerned the social stratification of the use and non-use of the phonologically variable /r/ in New York City spoken words such as "fourth" and "floor." Labov's reason for focusing on /r/ was that the presence or absence of /r/ in certain words was suspected to be indicative of a person's socioeconomic class: those who belong to higher socioeconomic classes were expected to use /r/ more frequently than those of lower socioeconomic classes. Labov collected speech samples from employees at three different department stores: Saks Fifth Avenue, Macy's, and S. Klein. These stores were carefully chosen because of their typical clientele's socioeconomic status: upper-middle class, middle class, and working class, respectively. Labov's results supported his hypothesis about differential use of /r/ by employees at the three stores.

The second wave of sociolinguistic analysis combined ethnographic research methods and quantitative methods, with the goal of marking group memberships based on language choices. Like the first wave, it focused on demographic categories (e.g., age, sex, socioeconomic class, and race), which have been shown to explain patterns of linguistic variation. One such example is the large-scale sociolinguistic ASL study conducted by Ceil Lucas, Robert Bayley, and Clayton Valli in 1995. The goal of the ASL study was to find internal and external constraints on ASL variations, comparing the factors relevant to sign languages with those identified and described in spoken languages. The language-internal constraints examined include grammatical category, preceding phonological environment, following phonological environment, and genre of text (conversation or narrative). The external constraints include the typical social factors in sociolinguistic studies of spoken languages: age, gender, social class, race, and region. One additional social factor was also included in this study: audiological status of informants and their parents.

The researchers visited eight different US cities where deaf schools were located: Bellingham, Washington; Fremont, California; Olathe, Kansas; Kansas City, Missouri; New Orleans, Louisiana; Staunton, Virginia; Frederick, Maryland; and Boston, Massachusetts. During their site visits, the researchers and their associates filmed and interviewed ASL informants at community centers and domestic settings. After completing the site visits, the research team returned to their bases to tabulate possible variations. One kind of variation the researchers examined was phonological, including signs with the ♩ handshape, and signs with citation form on the forehead compared to ones with lowered locations; looking at these features allowed the researchers to study metathesis, a transposition of phonological units in a sign, such as producing the sign DEAFix (shown in Figure 8.5) with movement from the ear to the chin or from the chin to the ear. The researchers also looked at syntactic variation (the presence or absence of subject pronouns), and lexical variation (phonologically unrelated variants for the same concept, as in the different signs for BIRTHDAY shown above in Figure 8.3). It was a very large undertaking. The study found that

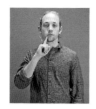

Figure 8.5 ASL sign DEAFix, with downward movement. Image: ASL Signbank, 2018.

ASL variation was defined by internal and external constraints similar to those identified as constraints in spoken languages, with the addition of audiological status, which is not typical in sociolinguistic studies of spoken languages.

One example of phonological feature variation studied by this group is the production of the sign DEAFix. Something as simple as signing DEAFix from ear to chin or chin to ear can be defined by geographic locations (Kansas/Missouri vs Massachusetts/Maryland) and age (young, middle age, and senior citizen). Variation in production of the sign DEAFix can also be explained by the immediate phonological environments, with the preceding or following signs influencing the movement direction of the sign from the top (if it follows a sign produced high on the head or precedes a sign produced low on the head) or below (vice versa).

So far, we have seen differences between middle-class and working-class speech, varieties explained by age and gender, and varieties accounted for by race and ethnicity. However, one critique of the first and second waves of sociolinguistic analysis is that the external factors are treated as though they are objective measures, but really they are socially constructed based on current ideologies. For example, gender, socioeconomic class, and race are historically treated as categorical, but people may not feel that they fully belong to one or another such category. For example, there are people who identify themselves based on a gender spectrum; this highlights that the socially imposed gender binary is not appropriate, and in fact, it may be harmful. Similarly, there are people born or brought into a certain socioeconomic class by their families or caregivers, but their own social networks with their peers are not always defined by their family's socioeconomic status. Multiracial and multiethnic identities are also on the rise, so separate racial and ethnic categories may not inform us of participants' language choices. Socially constructed categories can change with culture and time, so they should not be treated as objective measures.

In view of this changing approach to demographics, the third wave of sociolinguistic research considers communities of practice (CoP) as a factor in defining linguistic patterns and behaviors.

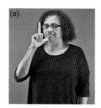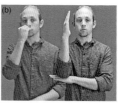

Figure 8.6 Variants of the ASL sign, LUNCH: (a) initialized variant with the 👋 handshape and (b) uninitialized variant EAT-NOON "lunch" with the 👌 and 👍 handshapes. Images: ASL Signbank, 2018.

Individuals regularly participate in social networks that are not readily explained by traditional demographic categories. Instead, their linguistic patterns and behaviors can be explained by their dynamic local group networks created and maintained by them at a given time and place. For example, Penelope Eckert did a study in 2000 on the social networks of high school students who called themselves "jocks" or "burnouts." Those who identified as jocks or burnouts could also be classified as middle-class and working-class groups, but the socioeconomic line was not that clear-cut because the students' social networks did not always mirror the social networks at home. Also, the high school students spent most of their time at school, where they frequently engaged in certain social groups, whether by choice or not, so it made sense to use their group memberships and their personal identities to explain the emergence and existence of linguistic differences, not the traditional social categories that are based on rigid notions.

The communities of practice approach can also apply to ASL and other sign languages. For example, signers involved in the ASL-centric movement are doing work to de-initialize signs that contain initialized handshapes (handshapes of the signs following the initial letter of English-equivalent words, as mentioned in Chapter 3, Section 3.2.3). They believe that those initialized signs are the result of English encroachment on ASL during the time that ASL was commonly believed to be a broken form of

English and was blamed for the English literacy problems that were common among deaf students. As an intervention to the literacy problem, a variety of English-based artificial systems of signs were created as an instructional method to support deaf children's English acquisition. But ASL is not the culprit for English literacy problems among deaf students; ASL is simply a different language from English. There are other factors contributing to literacy differences, including early language deprivation, access to English forms, reading resources and support, ideological differences in reading instruction, and so on. For these reasons, ASL centrists are fiercely protective of ASL and actively reject signs that have the appearance of influence from English. For example, the sign LUNCH is produced with the L handshape, 👆 (see Figure 8.6a). Signers who reject this version embrace a compound sign, EAT-NOON, which they deem to be conceptually accurate with the act of eating and the temporal depiction of noon, with no trace of English in the alternative form (see Figure 8.6b). ASL centrists even de-initialize signs by removing initialized handshapes in signs like FAMILY (see Figure 8.7) with the marked F handshape (👌) and replacing it with the "unmarked 5" handshape (🖐) that closes into the flat O handshape (👌). ASL centrists cannot easily be categorized by traditional social factors like sex, race, age, and occupation, but they can be defined by their ASL-centric language ideology of how ASL should be. By paying attention to their dynamic local networks, we could identify which groups or communities support the ASL-centric ideology and use such information for membership categories.

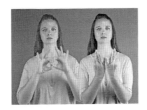

Figure 8.7 FAMILY with the 🖐 handshape. Image: ASL Signbank, 2018.

8.3.3 Factors unique to sign languages

Research shows that sign language varieties can be explained by external factors that include region, gender, age, ethnicity, and socioeconomic status. But due to the history of institutional and legal circumstances associated with educational and medical interventions related to deafness, we are compelled to include other factors that are not typical for variation in spoken languages. In particular, these factors concern how sign languages are transmitted in signing communities. We need to keep account of the language policies implemented in deaf education, the timing of children's access to sign language for its acquisition, the extent of sign language use at home (e.g., Deaf parents in an ASL-signing home vs. hearing parents in a nonsigning home), and the (additional) disabilities of signers (e.g., how Tactile ASL is used between DeafBlind signers).

Going back to the 1995 sociolinguistic study on ASL, Lucas, Bayley, and Valli showed a clear link between linguistic variation in ASL and the history of deaf education, in particular the language policies and programming at schools for the deaf through the 19th and 20th centuries. These policies ranged from the use of ASL in the classroom beginning in 1817 at the ASD, through the strict oralism that was enforced in most schools from the 1880s through the early 1970s (to the exclusion of sign language in the classroom), to the various "combined" methods of signing and talking simultaneously implemented in the 1970s, and finally back to the use of ASL in the classroom in many schools today. Educational and age factors contributing to linguistic varieties can be determined by federal policies on educational mainstreaming of disabled children and required accommodation in educational services. Before the 1960s, about 80% of deaf students in the United States attended specialized schools for the deaf. The specialized schools had resources to support the education of deaf children, whereas local schools in students' home districts did not have such resources available. By 2010, the percentage of deaf students attending specialized schools had declined to about 25%; many deaf students had the option of attending local schools where, by law or by choice, educational accommodations were provided to make it possible for them to receive education with their hearing peers.

Based on the history of educational and language policies in deaf education, Lucas, Bayley, and Valli found the age factor of their sign language informants to be an external constraint and grouped them into three generational age groups: 15–25, 26–54, and 55 and older. The age division followed the waves of language policies which the informants were subjected to as children. The Deaf informants in the group aged 55 and older were likely to be in deaf schools during the period when the speech-only policy was in effect. Nearly all deaf schools (except for black deaf schools) banned sign language in favor of the oral method. Despite the ban, deaf students discreetly used sign language among themselves out of instructors' and administrators' sight. The Deaf informants in the group aged 26–54 were likely to be instructed via the combined method of signing and speaking. In their lifetime, ASL was beginning to be recognized as a real language based on the serious linguistic inquiry by William Stokoe and his Deaf colleagues. At the same time, English-based sign communication codes were created as alternative signing methods to ASL, so that created a variety of communication experiences for this group of informants. The group of informants in the age group of 15–25 were educated at the time when ASL was accepted as the medium of instruction in classrooms and educational interpreters were available as part of the educational accommodation plan. The age division can be tied to legal developments in deaf education in the early 1970s with the passage of Public Law 94–142 (the Education of All Handicapped Children Act of 1975) and in the change of communication methods from oral to signed including ASL and English-based artificial systems. Similar educational developments can be found in other parts of the world. For example, in Italy, a similar trend emerged in the late 1970s with the passage of legislation on the mainstreaming of children with disabilities, including deaf and hard of hearing children. In New Zealand, the mainstream placement of deaf and hard of hearing children started to become common in the 1980s.

8.4 Impracticality of maintaining a universal sign language

There is one signed communication system that is designed to be accessible to signers of different nationalities in a cross-cultural setting: International Sign (IS). IS, like the invented spoken language Esperanto, is a flexible auxiliary code for people of different nationalities to communicate with each other without using their own languages. Users of IS can use a core common vocabulary, or their own signs from their native sign language if the signs' features are iconic or familiar enough to communicate intended meanings. The grammar of IS uses features that seem to be common across different sign languages, such as primarily following a topic-comment order and making use of spatial marking. Even though IS is of the signing modality and it has been used for decades, it is not considered by all to be a natural language according to the theoretical and evidence-based definitions of language. It is common to use the following properties as basic to a language: community conventions regulating the use and maintenance of symbols; relationships of symbols within a complex system; symbols that can be divided into discrete symbols; recursion with the strings of symbols; displacement strategies that refer to things and events outside of the immediate context; productivity, complexity, and creativity in using symbols and expressing information; transmission of language through generations within a community; and semantic and pragmatic contexts that infuse social meanings of the symbols. Even though studies on the linguistic features and structural analyses of IS are still in the early stage, at present it seems that IS satisfies some but not all of these properties. Furthermore, IS has its limitations when it comes to transmission and accessibility in the larger geographical regions.

IS is a context-dependent form of foreigner talk with a limited set of conventionalized signs that are combined with iconic signs borrowed from the users' sign languages. In some cases, IS heavily borrows signs from American- and European-based sign languages, depending on the communication context and the users' nationalities. There are anecdotal remarks regarding complaints about the encroachment of American- and European-based sign languages in IS, rendering it relatively inaccessible for people who are not familiar with American- and European-based sign languages. In either case with original or borrowed signs, IS is not available for every signer in the world, just as Esperanto is not available to every speaker. It is generally used by people who have means and privileges to travel, to engage in the international network as part of their occupations or hobbies, and to possess technological devices to communicate with people in different countries. The typical locales for IS as a communication for contact are conferences, organized sports competitions, tourism, or on social media where the intended audience includes people of different nationalities. For example, the World Federation of the Deaf (WFD), the World Association of Sign Language Interpreters (WASLI), and Theoretical Issues in Sign Language Research (TISLR) are international conferences hosted every few years. Presenters and attendees at these conferences often use IS when they engage in the professional network for sharing and discussing their works. Deaflympics, hosted by the International Committee of Sports for the Deaf (ICSD) as a governing body, is another venue where IS is used as a convenient contact communication system. It is a biennial sports event that alternates between winter and summer games, following the same format as the International Olympics but for athletes with qualified hearing loss and athletic skills. However, some athletes and spectators at the Deaflympics, just like attendees at professional conferences, may use their own sign languages and interpreters in case IS is not accessible to them. Note that these events are held every few years, so IS does not have a stable community in a physical habitat where members can use it as their primary means of communication.

IS is a useful communication tool for people who are familiar with it, but not for people who have never been or are rarely exposed to it. In a hypothetical case, if IS were adopted by a community in which every generation used it as their primary communication, IS would be conventionalized in a way that follows the properties of natural languages and it would be categorized as a sign language. Based on the definitions of language and the limitations of IS, we cannot say that a universal sign language truly exists. In reality, there are multiple sign languages that exist in different parts of the world along social and geographic lines, just as with spoken languages.

8.5 Conclusion

Theories of linguistic structure alone cannot account for all linguistic patterns and behaviors shown by human beings who speak or sign. The sociocultural aspect of language communities must be observed to understand how historical impacts and accidents define languages, and how geographical and social factors shape and maintain languages. Adding the social component to linguistic theories does not make them any less scientific. It enhances our understanding of language systems.

Discussion questions

1   What is the relationship between diglossia and domains?
2   What are the two main factors in language variation?
3   With so many variants in ASL, should standardization of ASL signs be the goal in deaf education and sign language interpreting programs? Why or why not?

Further reading

Eichmann, H., & Rosenstock, R. (2014). Regional variation in German Sign Language: the role of schools (re-)visited. *Sign Language Studies; Washington, 14*(2), 175–202.
This article examines the generational difference related to the role of deaf education in maintaining or changing variation in sign language.

Fenlon, J., & Wilkinson, E. (2015). Sign languages in the world. In A. C. Schembri & C. Lucas (Eds.), *Sociolinguistics and deaf communities* (pp. 5–28). Cambridge, England: Cambridge University Press.
This book chapter provides an overview of the current state of sign languages and their categorizations.

Langman, J. (2013). Analyzing qualitative data: mapping the research trajectory in multilingual contexts. In R. Bayley, R. Cameron, & C. Lucas (Eds.), *The Oxford handbook of sociolinguistics* (pp. 241–260). Oxford, England: Oxford University Press.
This book chapter provides an overview of the different phases of sociolinguistic analysis as discussed in the chapter.

Lucas, C., Bayley, R., & Valli, C. (2001). *Sociolinguistic variation in American Sign Language*. Washington, DC: Gallaudet University Press.
This book is a sociolinguistic study of ASL variation based on seven different sites in the United States.

McCaskill, C., Lucas, C., Bayley, R., & Hill, J. C. (2011). *The hidden treasure of Black ASL: its history and structure.* Washington, DC: Gallaudet University Press.
This book is a sociolinguistic study of Black ASL as a distinct dialect, which is defined by social and geographic constraints as discussed in the chapter.

Simons, G. F., & Fennig, C. D. (Eds.). (2018). *Ethnologue: languages of the world* (21st ed.). Dallas, TX: SIL International. https://www.ethnologue.com/
This resource contains a section on language families that include sign languages. It is available both in hard copy and online.

Bibliography

Geraci, C., Battaglia, K., Cardinaletti, A., Cecchetto, C., Donati, C., Giudice, S., & Mereghetti, E. (2011). The LIS corpus project: a discussion of sociolinguistic variation in the lexicon. *Sign Language Studies, 11*(4), 528–574.

LeMaster, B. (1999). Reappropriation of gendered Irish Sign Language in one family. *Visual Anthropology Review, 15*(2), 69–83.

Lucas, C., Bayley, R., McCaskill, C., & Hill, J. (2015). The intersection of African American English and Black American Sign Language. *International Journal of Bilingualism, 19*(2), 156–168.

McKee, R., & McKee, D. (2011). Old signs, new signs, whose signs? Sociolinguistic variation in the NZSL lexicon. *Sign Language Studies, 11*(4), 485–527.

Monaghan, L. (2003). A world's eye view: deaf cultures in global perspectives. In L. Monaghan, C. Schmaling, K. Nakamura, & G. H. Turner (Eds.), *Many ways to be deaf: international variation in deaf communities* (pp. 1–24). Washington, DC: Gallaudet University Press.

Padden, C. (2011). Sign language geography. In G. Mathur & D. J. Napoli (Eds.), *Deaf around the world: the impact of language* (pp. 19–37). Oxford, England: Oxford University Press.

Parisot, A. -M., Rinfret, J., Villeneueve, S., & Voghel, A. (2015). Quebec Sign Language/Langue des signes québécoise (LSQ). In J. B. Jepsen, G. de Clerck, S. Lutalo-Kiingi, & W. B. McGregor (Eds.), *Sign languages of the world: a comparative handbook* (pp. 701–728). Berlin, Germany: De Gruyter, Inc.

Rosenstock, R. (2008). The role of iconicity in International Sign. *Sign Language Studies, 8*(2), 131–159.

Schembri, A., & Johnson, T. (2013). Sociolinguistic variation and change in sign languages. In R. Bayley, R. Cameron, & C. Lucas (Eds.), *The Oxford handbook of sociolinguistics* (pp. 503–524). Oxford, England: Oxford University Press.

Stamp, R., Schembri, A., Fenlon, J., Rentelis, R., Woll, B., & Cormier, K. (2014). Lexical variation and change in British Sign Language. *PLoS One; San Francisco, 9*(4), e94053.

Van Herreweghe, M., & Vermeerbergen, M. (2009). Flemish Sign Language standardisation. *Current Issues in Language Planning, 10*(3), 308–326.

Wolfram, W., & Schilling, N. (2016). *American English, dialects and variation* (3rd ed.). Oxford, England: Wiley Blackwell.

Chapter 9

Language attitudes

9.1 Defining attitudes

Attitudes are part of how we think and believe. They are part of how we act. They are part of how we feel. An attitude is a psychological tendency in our reaction to an object we favor or disfavor. There are three components of attitudes: cognitive, affective, and behavioral, and they may not be harmonious; they can exist in conflict with each other. For example, we can hate Spongebob Squarepants with little knowledge of the character, yet we might tolerate him because we don't want to offend our friend who is a fan of Spongebob Squarepants. This is something we do all the time. It influences our interactions with each other, shapes our views of the world, and regulates how we feel about a particular object, be it tangible or intangible. This object is called an *attitude object*. In the example above, Spongebob Squarepants is an attitude object toward which we direct our thoughts, feelings, and behaviors. As with any part of our selves, attitudes change. If we understand why Spongebob Squarepants is the way he is with his annoyingly sunny view on life and his loveable awkward personality, our feelings toward him may change, and we too might become a fan of Spongebob Squarepants. Anything can be an attitude object and it can be tangible or intangible. In the case under consideration, language can be an attitude object toward which we express positive or negative attitudes. Furthermore, our attitudes are always tied to social advantages or disadvantages, and this has an impact on language as well.

9.2 Attitudes toward language, culture, and identity

At some point, we may have heard or uttered statements like *French sounds sexy, Italian is full of passion, British English sounds proper, German sounds pushy, Arabic sounds scary,* or *American English sounds casual.* The statements may feel true to us based on our perception of how the speech sounds to us, but such statements are tied to the stereotypes we have gleaned from experience, media, and conversation, and not the inherent linguistic truth about languages. These languages are just rule-based systems of symbols that happen to be spoken. We give them context based on what we think and know about them and their language communities, including stereotypes that have been impressed on us. Sign languages are also subjected to this kind of perception as well whether we know them or not: *American Sign Language is beautiful to look at, British Sign Language looks cool with the two-handed alphabet, Japanese Sign Language looks awkward but unique,* and *Italian Sign Language looks like it is full of passion.* Again, these statements are not inherently true. Sign languages are also rule-based systems of symbols that happen to be signed. We create a reality about sign languages based on what we think they are, factually or otherwise. Language is not just a rule-based communication tool; it is also a cultural tool and it serves as a cultural marker of a language community that is subject to judgments from society.

9.2.1 The case of racism and language in the United States

African American English (AAE) is one of the dialects that is stigmatized based on racial and linguistic differences. In the United States, the history of racism has left its marks everywhere, including on English. AAE is just like any language variety, that is, a complex and organized system of symbols regulated by community conventions, but because of its association with black Americans, it often elicits negative responses and stereotypes. Elsewhere, AAE is considered hip or cool, such as in the entertainment industry, but it is also publicly mocked or criticized on social and news media platforms for its linguistic differences. Black actors are typically cast in stereotypical and unflattering roles as criminals, victims, or servants that require them to speak AAE as a way to be "authentically black or ethnic." In education, black children who use AAE tend to be perceived as linguistically incompetent and may be improperly diagnosed as having a learning disability or speech impediment. Just imagine how teachers come to that conclusion when they hear children saying these sentences: *"Who dat?"*, *"Where you at?"*, *"Stop keep axing me"*, *"She don't know"*, *"Imma go to a libary"*, and *"He finna go to the bafroom."* In those AAE sentences, the phonological, morphological, and syntactical structures are quite regular. If AAE is the only language used at the students' home and in their neighborhood, that is their main linguistic exposure and they use it as such. To the teachers who don't have basic linguistic knowledge, the students simply speak incorrectly, when in fact, they simply don't have consistent exposure to Mainstream American English (MAE) to acquire as a second dialect.

In the mid-1990s, a public school in Oakland, California, implemented a program for black children to use AAE as an instructional method, in a similar vein as a bilingual education program. In the Oakland program, two different English varieties, AAE and MAE, were used to reinforce the students' academic learning. The news of the bidialectal education program resulted in a public outcry that called for its end. As a dutiful response to the outcry, the Linguistic Society of America (LSA), the professional organization of academics and researchers to support advancement in the scientific study of languages, issued a resolution in 1997 to clarify that AAE was a valid dialect as a rule-based system with regular linguistic expressions. They also explained that the controversy surrounding stigmatized languages and dialects was more based on social and political grounds than linguistic grounds.

Despite the intervention from the LSA, linguistic discrimination and oppression continues with the American collective psyche steeped in a history of racism along with misconceptions about how language works. For example, linguistic profiling, studied by a sociolinguist named John Baugh, occurs in the case of housing discrimination against black Americans based on their speech alone. It can take just a single word, "hello," for a housing agent to identify a caller's race. The Fair Housing Act (FHA) prohibits blatant racial discrimination in housing sales and rentals, but it is difficult to prove a racial intent in the denial of sales or rental housing because of linguistic profiling. If the discrimination is based on the color of the applicant's skin, the case is clear-cut because racial minorities are under the protection clause and swift actions will be taken; but when apparent discrimination is based on speech, racial intent is not as easily proven, and furthermore, language itself is not under the protection clause. For example, if a black person uses racially marked speech in a phone call with a landlord and requests an appointment for an apartment visit, the landlord may say it is not available when, in fact, it is. If the black caller suspects the landlord's racial intent in the denial of rental housing, the caller can call again with a "professional" voice in MAE making the same request and suddenly the apartment is available for a visit. If that black caller shows up to visit, the landlord will see the person and apologize profusely about the wasted visit now that the apartment is not available anymore. The burden is on the caller to collect evidence of racial discrimination since the landlord has not explicitly said anything about race and has been polite on the phone and in person. Linguistic profiling is not limited to housing discrimination. It is also a problem in employment, education, and the legal system, where racial intent is also harder to prove.

In Chapter 8, we discussed how racial segregation affected the formation of Black American Sign Language (ASL) at the Southern schools for black Deaf children prior to the landmark 1954 Supreme Court case, *Brown v. Board of Education of Topeka*. Under the state sanctioned segregation policy, black Deaf students had virtually no contact with white Deaf students, and black and white schools were completely separated. That included educational facilities, resources, and sign languages. Former Deaf students of segregated black schools often remarked that they could not understand the signing of white Deaf students and teachers, so that suggests a significant amount of vocabulary difference and distinct language practices between southern black and white Deaf communities. During the process of desegregation, black Deaf students were transferred to white deaf schools and they were left to navigate a new linguistic landscape with the signing of white Deaf peers and white educators and administrators. As is true for every state with a history of segregation, the education of black and white students was not equal in terms of resources, facilities, and quality, so when black Deaf students saw that white deaf schools had better facilities and services, they naturally determined that their old schools were not of superior quality. Because of this, Black Deaf students assumed that their own signing was inferior to that of white signers. Their assumption was based on the difficulty in understanding the signing of white peers and adults, which led the black students to reason that the white signing was more advanced, with a more extensive vocabulary, complex grammar, and a specific signing style. In reality, of course, the language was simply new to them; their Black ASL was a valid, rule-governed language and it had worked for them prior to desegregation. It was unfortunate that they were led to feel ashamed of their own language.

Today, the older version of Black ASL that developed at the former black deaf schools remains with the aging population of black Deaf people and their families, and that puts their variety in an endangered status. Black Deaf students currently acquire the mainstream dialect of ASL at their schools and they have little or no access to the former signing of aging black Deaf signers. Despite the loss of distinct vocabulary, there still exists a black cultural basis that stylistically defines the Black ASL variety with differences in phonology, morphology, vocabulary, and discourse, particularly with lexical borrowing from AAE. In the current generation of black Deaf signers, some have expressed a black cultural pride in their marked differences in signing, but some still have internalized negative messages about such differences, qualifying them with terms having negative connotations: "thuggish," "street," or "ghetto." This indicates how powerful stigmatization works in coloring the perception of language that stems from our unconscious racial bias.

9.2.2 The case of cultural identity and language in the American Deaf community

Hearing people who have had no association with Deaf people or have not taken sign language classes are largely ignorant about sign language. As discussed in Chapter 8, they may mistakenly assume that sign language is universal around the world and believe that Deaf people of different nationalities can communicate with one another effortlessly.

Another mistaken belief is that sign language is a visual representation of the spoken language of the country, but again this is not the case. Sign languages are structurally different from spoken languages in many ways. We can see that this is so because alternative artificial systems have been developed in order to represent spoken languages manually. For example, Signing Exact English (SEE) was invented as one of several artificial systems to represent English during the 1970s. SEE was designed as a replacement for ASL in school to teach English to deaf students. SEE was easier to acquire than ASL for educators and administrators, who were typically hearing English speakers, because English was their primary language and they only needed to learn signs to match with English words, and sign them in English structure. But for Deaf students, English in the auditory form was not easily accessible for them, so they did not pick it up at home or in school, so SEE in the visual form was not a simple mapping. SEE is furthermore too unnatural and cumbersome for children to pick up regular linguistic patterns, and moreover, not all adults were consistent or proficient in the use of SEE. But if SEE was the only exposure they had in their childhood, it was their primary communication tool and they had to make do with what communication and language input they could get. As a result, it made their signing different from their peers who acquired ASL as their natural language.

The use of ASL is one of the qualifications that signals a cultural membership in the Deaf community, along with other properties and artifacts such as sign names, sense of community, shared values and customs, cultural knowledge, history, social structure, and arts. Even Deaf children are aware of cultural identities based on language use, and they tend to socialize with others who are most like them language-wise, for example, including those who are proficient in ASL and excluding those who are less proficient. There is even a perception of a standard variety of ASL. The earliest recognition of a standard ASL dialect can be dated back to 1834, which is around the time when a number of deaf schools were founded and operated with sign language, having been transmitted from the first public school for deaf students in Hartford, Connecticut. When Gallaudet College (now Gallaudet University) was founded in 1864, Deaf graduates from the schools continued their education and maintained their language variety on campus. Naturally, the ASL variety at Gallaudet acquired prestige based on the privileged access to educational and professional networks that Gallaudet graduates enjoyed. Over decades, the community's cultural wealth had been steadily building with ASL as its linguistic capital at Gallaudet and elsewhere. What followed was a gatekeeping mechanism for those who were included in or excluded from the Deaf community based on the use of ASL and access to community networks and the kind of signing or communication preference as a perceived marker of cultural identity: ASL as a social marker for people who are involved in the Deaf community; SEE as a social marker for people who are not as involved in the Deaf community; and a mixture of ASL and Signed English as a social marker for people in between the Deaf and hearing worlds. Individuals with hearing loss have a personal, albeit difficult, journey to portray what kind of deaf people they want to be based on the intersection of multiple identities and contexts.

9.3 Notion of standard and prestige

A language variety, be it language or dialect, that has been widely used in a society may come to be viewed as standard in the sense of "proper" or correct. Such a view influences speakers' ideology of what language is and how it is supposed to be used. If the ideology is very powerful, that may make the community want to defend their language by keeping it pure and defending its correctness. But purity and correctness do not apply to languages, which are naturally constantly changing and responding to various conditions. By what benchmark would a language be judged pure and correct? If there is a benchmark, does it apply to everyone in the community or only to certain groups of people? What or who determines these requirements?

9.3.1 Linguistic and social differences between varieties

The perception of standard and stigmatized languages is explained by social advantages or disadvantages that exist in the society. To understand how the language judgment benchmark works based on linguistic purity and correctness, Figure 9.1 illustrates how language varieties differentiate based on prestige and stigma. Varieties A, B, and C are dialects of the same language and varieties D and E are two different languages. We can see that variety C occupies the highest status. Variety C is buoyed by social prestige that is recognized and desired by everyone. It is used everywhere so it is perceived as standard and judged to be correct and pure. Variety B does share some structure with C, but its linguistic difference lessens its desirability and it is judged to be less correct, but variety A has even more undesirable features and they reduce its desirability as a stigmatized variety. As for the

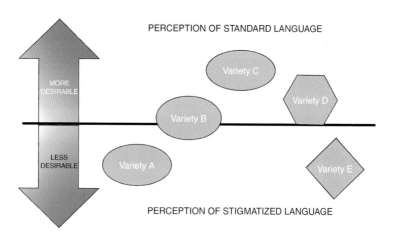

Figure 9.1 A schematic diagram of language varieties from the social view.

other languages, varieties D and E are in two different positions: D is in a favorable position with desirable features and E is in an unfavorable position with its stigmatized features. Even though D is in the favorable position like C, C is the most favorable one due to its power, presence, and history.

In Figure 9.2, it is a different story. All languages and dialects are equally valid as rule-based linguistic systems. From the linguistic perspective, we look at the linguistic structure of language varieties and describe them as they are. If they are similar in structure, we look for linguistic, social, and historical factors that explain the similarities. Whether one variety is better than the others is not the overall goal in the study of linguistics. The first three varieties, A, B, and C, are grouped together based on lexical and structural similarities and mutual intelligibility, as illustrated by the use of the same shape. Based on this fact, we can determine that they are dialects. Possible explanations for the similarities could be a political history of colonization or secession, geographical barriers in the region that isolate the language communities, or a cultural difference between the language communities based on social and religious practices. Varieties D and E are two different languages based on their

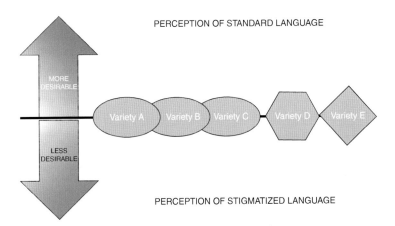

Figure 9.2 A schematic diagram of language varieties from the linguistic view.

linguistic structures and cultural histories. They are not mutually intelligible with each other and with the other varieties. In addition to linguistic analysis, we can refer to geographic and social factors to explain the similarities and differences between the varieties without judging their intrinsic or social worth. That is the difference between understanding the comparative structure of the varieties and believing some varieties are better or worse than others.

9.3.2 Overt prestige

No language variety is inherently better than another, but communities do assign positive and negative social values to them, which mark some varieties as standard and others as stigmatized. A standard language variety acquires prestige when it is associated with a community of individuals with desirable traits, typically in the form of social, economic, educational, and political advantages. Over time, the language variety becomes deeply entrenched in the community so that it is recognized as part of the institution in every way. Naturally, it is seen as a legitimate and recognizable language in a greater community.

For example, in the United States, English is the standard language, despite the fact that it has not been recognized as an official language by law, and the fact that the country has at least 350 languages used at home, including sign languages. But not all languages are stigmatized by default. French, Italian, and German spoken on US soil may be regarded as different though acceptable or desirable, but Spanish, Arabic, and Navajo receive markedly negative attention due to the history of racism, xenophobia, and anti-immigration sentiments – despite the fact that Navajo is indigenous to the country. English has several different dialects spoken in the country, but the MAE dialect is the rule in education, workplaces, media, and government. Certain accents are acceptable as standard, but if stigmatized accents are used, the users will receive unwanted negative attention.

ASL is markedly different from English in both its signed mode and as a linguistic system. It is associated with individuals with hearing disability, which is generally undesirable because it is not part of the social norm. But interestingly enough, ASL is seen as desirable outside of the United States. The country is historically seen as the land of opportunity and a safe destination for people emigrating from developing and underdeveloped countries or from countries in political or violent conflict. The positive values that are assigned to the United States lend themselves to the prestigious languages that happen to include ASL on this view. Historically, ASL was imported to other countries through missionaries, developmental work, or educational advancement and it came to be viewed as desirable because it was presented as a better, or in some cases only, choice, whether or not sign languages existed in these areas before the arrival of ASL. This has happened in some African countries, Puerto Rico, Thailand, Japan, and many others.

A language that is perceived to be standard carries an *overt prestige*, a form of acknowledgment with the sense of correctness based on the language's association with greater social, economic, educational, and political benefits. There is no inherent value since the language is basically a rule-based communication tool for a community to use. The social benefits extend to the language based on its association with a community of privileged individuals. Those individuals live, breathe, and consume the language every day of their lives until the language is culturally bound to them. As with any tool, the language can in principle be used by outsiders or people with less privilege if they know how to use it, and the privilege associated with it may extend success to them depending on how well they fit in. For example, college-educated people from a working poor background may sound like they are from a metropolitan city, especially if they try to hide their working-class accent. AAE speakers sound "white" when they switch to MAE when talking with white people. Chief executive officers (CEOs) who are women may speak like men in an assertive style if they command respect from them. Deaf signers will have to modify their signing in a manner that follows the structure of spoken language if they want to be accepted as equals among hearing speakers. Had any of these individuals refused to make a linguistic choice to use a standard variety, they would be at a disadvantage, depending on the circumstances.

9.3.3 Covert prestige

A language associated with communities with lesser social, economic, educational, and political benefits in society is perceived to be stigmatized. Stigmatized communities are historically or institutionally marginalized in a way that distances them from privileged communities. The distance can be any form of social or geographic barrier as we have discussed in the previous chapter. With the barriers and the ideology that have been shaped and defined by the use of standard language, negative attitudes are formed and maintained in society. Negative attitudes are typically expressed by privileged communities that carry negative opinions and beliefs about other communities. Negative attitudes can be internalized by members of the marginalized communities experiencing institutional and personal treatment they have received throughout their lives. This is called *linguistic insecurity*. That, in turn, can affect how they maintain their own language varieties.

For example, at some point in Hawaii, university students of Japanese ancestry expressed that as children they felt embarrassed about speaking Japanese and felt pressured to conform by using English with their American peers. They were a linguistic minority and they didn't want to appear different from their peers. They didn't understand the necessity of using their native language, but as adults, they understood and embraced the cultural and familial values of the language, maintaining Japanese as part of their cultural identity. Unfortunately for some of them, they were not as fluent in Japanese. This was the price they paid for being linguistically insecure. Another example is in Flanders, Belgium, where there are five different dialects of Flemish Sign Language (VGT, 'Vlaamse Gebarentaal') produced by five different deaf schools in the regions, which is typical. Deaf Belgians are used to such variation and they manage to understand each other in a communication situation, but at some point in the history, the signing diversity presented a problem for hearing people who were not fluent in VGT. As a response to the problem, a language standardization project was begun to develop Signed Dutch, an artificial sign system of Dutch, in a similar manner as Signed English in place of ASL in the United States. Signed Dutch was much easier for hearing people to acquire, but its structure was

different from VGT, which was already a full-fledged language for
Deaf Belgians. Because of Signed Dutch's association with Dutch
as a standard language and its use by hearing people, it acquired
social prestige and this resulted in Deaf Belgians' experience of
linguistic insecurity.

Despite linguistic insecurity, marginalized language communities can be protective of their own language and maintain it as a
badge of solidarity among themselves. Within their communities,
they view and treat each other favorably based on their use of
language that is different from the standard of the prestige community. The desire to belong in a community and the desire to be
authentic take precedence over social stigma based on language
use; this is described as *covert prestige*. Overt prestige describes a
broad acknowledgment of language as a status symbol whereas
covert prestige describes a sense of acceptance and belonging
based on the authentic knowledge or mastery of a stigmatized
language. If an outsider cannot master the stigmatized language,
the person would experience some form of isolation or exclusion
in the community whether the person is of the same cultural background or not.

For example, Jamaican Creole is stigmatized because it is considered "unclean" and it is associated with social, moral, and political degradation, despite the fact that it is the language of the
Jamaican community. Jamaican creole speakers uphold English
as a standard language, which is attributed to the history of colonization. Despite their own linguistic insecurity about Jamaican
Creole, they still speak creole with each other outside of school
and work to maintain social connection and belonging. Jamaican
recording artists still sing in Jamaican Creole to remain authentic and connect with their audience. Even teachers speak creole
with each other casually, although they may still proclaim that
they speak English all the time. If an American with no Jamaican
ancestry lives on the island and wants to connect with them, the
American will try to adopt the creole as one of their dialects in order to be welcomed into the community. However, if a Jamaican
citizen refuses to speak Jamaican creole based on the belief that
English is superior, the person risks being socially ostracized on
the basis of implicit social attitudes against the Jamaican community. That's one social privilege that this citizen has lost as a

Jamaican islander. If this same person doesn't master mainstream English with the appropriate accent, word choice, and sentence structure, it would be difficult for the person to gain the same privilege as fluent English speakers have. That's a double loss of privilege for the person who does not accept Jamaican Creole as a valid linguistic system and who is not as proficient in the standard English dialect.

Covert prestige is also present in the case of sign languages although they are typically stigmatized in most of the world due to the difference in modality and linguistic structure. As mentioned earlier in the chapter, we know that ASL was not accepted as a valid language in the education context and several versions of Signed English were designed as replacement visual communication systems for Deaf students. For decades, Deaf students internalized the message that ASL was not as good as English and hearing teachers and administrators maintained that message through instruction and school policy. Despite their linguistic insecurity, Deaf students still used ASL among themselves. Because hearing teachers and administrators were not interested in learning ASL, they would miss the inside information that ASL signers shared with each other, so the students took advantage of their ignorance. This is a form of covert prestige. Suppose that a student preferred to use Signed English instead of ASL and judged ASL to be inferior, that student would be favored by the teachers and administrators, but the ASL signing peers wouldn't be as friendly with the student. If social isolation bothered the student more than being a teacher's favorite, the student would acquire ASL to the fullest and eventually be welcomed into the fold with their ASL peers. This is not to say that people have to abandon one variety for another for the purpose of gaining overt or covert privilege. People can use multiple language forms in different settings and with different people to achieve different kinds of desired connections.

9.4 Language attitudes and choices in a diglossic context

In a diglossic situation, people always employ different strategies to portray their social identities, manage their language proficiencies, and reveal or withhold their language ideology. Consciously or unconsciously, they make a linguistic choice based on these questions: "How do I want to be treated?" "Who do I want to be?" "How can I get them to trust me?" "Is it safe to do this?" "What will I gain or lose if I do this?" and so on. For every question, the answer depends on the history and culture of the community, community privileges that individuals have, and social differences and geographic distances between groups of individuals.

Earlier in the chapter, we discussed the case of linguistic profiling of AAE speakers. AAE is usually spoken within informal community domains among black Americans. Not all black Americans speak AAE nor is AAE exclusive to black Americans. As with any variety, anyone can acquire it as long as they have access and exposure to it. When they use AAE outside of their community, they risk being judged for using a variety that is perceived to be inappropriate and unprofessional. If they want to avoid judgment and gain favor, they code-switch to MAE. *Code-switching* is a practice of alternating between two or more language varieties within a single encounter and it can include a single word, a sentence, or the entire conversation. So if an AAE speaker communicates with an MAE speaker, the AAE speaker may feel uncomfortable using AAE lest the MAE speaker cast judgment based on their language use. The AAE speaker will code-switch to MAE and remain there until they complete their conversation. When the AAE speaker recognizes a friend who also speaks AAE, the speaker will feel more comfortable and safe to switch back into AAE. They could communicate in MAE but unless they are in a formal domain, they are less motivated to do so due to covert prestige. If both of them have mastered AAE and MAE, they may use sentence-internal code-switching, depending on the domains they are in.

Code-switching is also practiced in signing communities depending on social and linguistic domains. As discussed earlier in the chapter, in the 20th century, American deaf schools enforced a form of language policy that ranged from a total ban of sign language to using English-based artificial sign systems as a replacement for ASL (see also Chapter 10 on language policy). If Deaf students violated the policy by using ASL, they would face consequences, especially during the oralism period when Deaf students received corporal punishment or had their hands tied for signing. Such punishment was discontinued later in the century, but some form of discouragement remained due to the language ideology. The language policy created a diglossic situation in which Deaf students would comply with the teachers' language by speaking or signing English in the classroom and code-switch to ASL whenever and wherever they were unsupervised. Through education, the students internalized such values about English and ASL during their years of school based on teachers' attitudes, and they maintained the code-switching practice throughout their lifetime.

In 1989, a language attitude study was done with student teachers who were still in deaf education training. Student teachers were asked to rate ASL and Signed English samples as part of the study. The result was that the teachers highly favored Signed English over ASL. Even though they rated ASL as more expressive, exciting, and faster, they saw Signed English as a better choice because they perceived it to be more precise, complete, consistent, and functional. As a language, ASL can be those things as well but it is not ideologically aligned with English. In the same year, another study was carried out to investigate sociolinguistic and communication profiles and attitudes of Deaf college students. Deaf college students who had a strong tie to Deaf culture highly favored ASL over English, but students who were hard of hearing or oral favored English (spoken or signed) over ASL. Ironically, even with the positive support of ASL from culturally Deaf students, ASL was still seen as a broken form of English with improper grammar and the attitude was that English speech must be taught in order for Deaf students to fit in with the larger society. ASL was also perceived to be associated with a lower education level as opposed to English, which was associated with a higher education level.

A lot has changed since 1989. Deaf cultural pride has been gaining steam with ASL and cultural materials available in publications, media, and online resources. ASL is more accepted in its current form and English-based artificial systems of signs are not as embraced as they were decades earlier. In 2010, a research study reassessed the Deaf community's attitudes toward ASL and Signed English. Deaf participants were asked to categorize different language samples with varying amounts of ASL and English features, from ones with more ASL features to ones with more English features. The samples also contained *contact signing*, which is a mixture of ASL and English features. Nearly all participants made similar categorizations of the signing samples based on the amount of ASL and English features: *ASL, contact signing*, and *Signed English* (see the video examples on the companion website, 9.1–9.4). After categorizing the samples, they were asked to evaluate the language characteristics and the personality of the signers in the signing samples. Based on the results, ASL was generally favored across the board and English was disfavored. Education was no longer a strong indicator for the prestige of ASL and English. The stigma of ASL has lessened so that now ASL can be used in formal domains.

A diglossic situation doesn't have to be limited to spoken-to-spoken language and spoken-to-sign-languages; it can include sign-to-sign languages. For example, in Mali of West Africa, Malian Sign Language (LSM) and ASL exist in diglossia with ASL as the most prestigious language. The Malian Deaf community recognizes the educational value of ASL because it is used as the medium of instruction in deaf education. Due to its lack of presence in education, LSM is perceived as stigmatized. However, a current language project is documenting the linguistic structure of LSM as a way to combat the stigma, so the diglossic situation may change eventually.

9.5 Conclusion

It is important to understand that there is no intrinsic differential of worth in language varieties due to their linguistic distinctions. As varieties meet all of the properties that define a language, they are equally valid as languages. The perceived differences in their linguistic value are tied to social values assigned by those outside the communities. The social values are defined by geographic, social, and historical factors that either elevate or lower their cultural worth and this influences how people from different language communities behave with each other. But over time, language worth changes along with cultural and political changes as we can see in the case of ASL. It used to be heavily stigmatized but with the increasing awareness of its true linguistic nature and the cultural impact from the Deaf community on the public, the language status of ASL is more secure now. In the next chapter, we see how language status is also affected with the help of language policy and planning.

Discussion questions

1   Define "attitude object" and explain its meaning with the example of language as an attitude object.
2   What is the difference between overt prestige and covert prestige?
3   In your experience, can you identify a form of diglossia in your life?
4   In your opinion, what factors influence code-switching?

Further reading

Baugh, J. (2007). Attitudes toward variations and ear-witness testimony: Linguistic profiling and voice discrimination in the quest for fair housing and fair lending. In R. Bayley & C. Lucas (Eds.), *Sociolinguistic variation: theories, methods, and applications* (pp. 338–348). Cambridge, England: Cambridge University Press.
This book chapter explores the concepts of linguistic profiling and how a voice identification can be the basis of discrimination in the fair housing cases.

Bayley, R., Hill, J., Lucas, C., & McCaskill, C. (2018). Perceptions of Black American Sign Language. In B. E. Evans, E. J. Benson, & J. N. Stanford (Eds.), *Language regard: methods, variation and change* (pp. 167–182). Cambridge, England: Cambridge University Press.
This book chapter presents different factors that explain the perceptions of Black ASL from black Deaf signers.

Hill, J. C. (2012). *Language attitudes in the American deaf community.* Washington, DC: Gallaudet University Press.

This book includes a comprehensive review of language attitude studies and empirical study of language perception and attitudes in the American Deaf community with respect to signing variation.

Krausneker, V. (2015). Ideologies and attitudes toward sign languages: an approximation. *Sign Language Studies*, *15*(4), 411.
This article reviews the categories of ideological constructions that influence attitudes toward sign languages.

Nyst, V. (2015). The sign language situation in Mali. *Sign Language Studies; Washington*, *15*(2), 126–150.
This article describes the sign language situation in Mali, specifically the diglossic function of Mali Sign Language and American Sign Language.

Bibliography

Eichmann, H. (2009). Planning sign languages: Promoting hearing hegemony? Conceptualizing sign language standardization. *Current Issues in Language Planning*, *10*(3), 293–307.

Fontana, S., Corazza, S., Braem, P. B., & Volterra, V. (2017). Language research and language community change: Italian Sign Language, 1981–2013. *Sign Language Studies; Washington*, *17*(3), 363–398.

Garrett, P. (2010). *Attitudes to language*. Cambridge, England: Cambridge University Press.

Kannapell, B. (1989). An examination of deaf college students' attitudes toward ASL and English. In C. Lucas (Ed.), *The sociolinguistics of the deaf community* (pp. 191–210). San Diego, CA: Academic Press.

Nakamura, K. (2006). Creating and contesting signs in contemporary Japan: language ideologies, identity, and community in flux. *Sign Language Studies; Washington*, *7*(1), 11–29,102.

Purnell, T., Idsardi, W., & Baugh, J. (1999). Perceptual and phonetic experiments on American English dialect identification. *Journal of Language and Social Psychology*, *18*(1), 10–30.

Slegers, C. (2010). Signs of change: contemporary attitudes to Australian Sign Language. *Australian Review of Applied Linguistics*, *33*(1), 5.

Tamene, E. H. (2018). *The sociolinguistics of Ethiopian Sign Language: a study of language use and attitudes*. Washington, DC: Gallaudet University Press.

Ward Trotter, J. (1989). An examination of language attitudes of teachers of the deaf. In C. Lucas (Ed.), *The sociolinguistics of the deaf community* (pp. 211–228). San Diego, CA: Academic Press.

Wassink, A. B. (1999). Historic low prestige and seeds of change: attitudes toward Jamaican Creole. *Language in Society, 28*(1), 57–92.

Chapter 10

Language policy and planning

10.1 Written and unwritten rules for language use

We instinctively know how to use the different languages and dialects at our command depending on where we are and who we are with. Education can be a factor in how we use language, but it is not the only one. Family as an institution is another factor that influences how we use language. Language use depends on the neighborhood where we grew up, where we work, where we socialize, and many other factors. Any place where we use our language has written or (more often) unwritten rules for how language should be used and the consequences we will experience if we don't follow the rules of the community. We know better than to use profanity in the presence of someone honorable, but many of us can freely curse with our friends. Perhaps we can comfortably use Spanish in a multilingual neighborhood, but not in a monolingual neighborhood where antagonism against non-English languages is running high. African American English (AAE) speakers switch to Mainstream American English to accommodate their white customers at the workplace and switch back to AAE when they are among themselves. An ASL teacher might require all students to sign all the time in class without using their voice and punish students who violate the instructor's "no voice'" policy. Those language practices are regulated by explicit or implicit agreements we hold at the personal, community, and institutional levels. This is what we consider language policy.

Language policy has three different components: language practices with linguistic behaviors and choices in a community; beliefs and ideology about language and language use; and efforts in intervening, planning, or managing language practices. These components sometimes overlap, so that even though we can discuss them separately, they do inform one another.

10.2 Language practices

Language practices are what we are doing with our language in a particular setting with one or more people. The list of language practices is endless: having a heart-to-heart conversation with a friend, calling a customer service office, ordering at a restaurant, giving a presentation at a conference, reporting news, interviewing for a job, commanding people to do things, greeting customers at a store, singing a song, reading a book, writing an email, interpreting for a client, and so on.

10.2.1 Language practices in sign language

Signers are typically bilingual in sign and spoken languages. Through experience and policy, teachers and students have developed the language practices that make their communication engagements possible. To have effective communication in the classroom, the teacher has to take a sign-centric approach to make sure that all participants are within each other's visual field in the physical space as they carry on a conversation. For example, the students typically sit around an arc or a circle so they can see each other. If the students sit in rows, they will have trouble seeing other students' signing and repeatedly adjust themselves in their seats to catch each other's comments. The teacher has to be in front of the class to stay within the students' visual field. If the teacher walks among the students in the classroom, it will compromise students' communication access, so it is better for the teacher to remain in front of the classroom. If the teacher needs to get full attention from distracted students, there are different ways to get attention: flashing the ceiling lights, waving the hands, or placing two 🖐 hands on both sides of the forehead as if signing ANTLERS (see Figure 10.1) and waiting for them to follow suit.

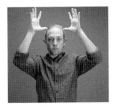

Figure 10.1 ASL sign, ANTLERS. Image: ASL Signbank, 2018.

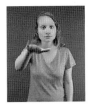

Figure 10.2 ASL sign, I(hey). Image: ASL Signbank, 2018.

If a student wants to get the attention of the teacher or a fellow student, the appropriate way is to tap on the shoulder or do a hand wave (see Figure 10.2) until the student gets their attention. There are other ways to get someone's attention such as shouting, whooping, stomping on the floor, or throwing a random object in their direction, but those behaviors are considered inappropriate at school. On the other hand, signers may engage in such behaviors naturally at home depending on the established practices of their families. In the classroom, the teacher and students may use an academic register of sign language. What is an appropriate academic register varies depending on the school, but commonly includes: using appropriate vocabulary and avoiding slang or profanity, minding body posture as one signs, mastering the communication discourse format in order to be clear to the audience, and polishing signed texts in a live or video presentation.

Business is another example that has its own language practices. Deaf people can conduct business with their colleagues and customers in sign language. If they have a meeting, they typically prefer to sit at a circular or oval table so they can see each other clearly; if the table is rectangular, people on the same side of the table would have more trouble following their side mates than they do with people across the table. If they need to make a phone call, the signers can use a specialized videophone with standalone hardware or as an app on a mobile device. It is similar to FaceTime or Skype except that it is designed as a videophone device specifically for sign language interpreting service, along with technical support. Deaf people are typically bilingual, so they can follow the news in written or signed format; but if they prefer the latter, they have access to online news, for example, Daily Moth, Sign1News, D-Pan TV, and H3World TV. Those news services are designed to be culturally compatible with the signing audience's language reception with less distracting visual elements.

As with all languages, people are aware of the explicit and implicit language practices within their own communities; however, in a cross-intercultural interaction, conflicts are to be expected when people are not familiar with each other's cultural customs. For example, if a nonsigning teacher is not familiar with the classroom practices described above, the teacher would not manage the classroom effectively and the signing students would be disengaged. Unfortunately, this is a reality for many Deaf people who have experienced being in a classroom that is not sign-centric; this has been common for decades. Deaf students have had to develop various strategies to cope with inaccessible communication, which would not be necessary had teachers been more sensitive and accommodating to the students' communication and language needs. In all communication situations, we more or less have different scripts that help or hurt us when we navigate through different discourses in our languages. The scripts are shaped by language ideologies that we acquire, maintain, and change throughout our lifetimes.

10.3 Language ideology

Language ideology is a system of ideas that forms a basis for language practices among people in a community. Humans are incredibly diverse in their thinking and experiences, so the convergence and divergence of their ideas make a complex reality for those who believe what they know to be true about languages and people who use them. For example, in Montreal, Quebec, French and English have been part of Quebec citizens' lives so they expect to see both languages being used anywhere in the city. If someone from England moves to Montreal and opens an English-only restaurant with all menus in English, and they hire monolingual English-speaking employees, the restaurant will not last long in the city where the French-speaking community fought to receive respect for their language. Bilingualism is the rule. If that English restaurant owner moves to an English-speaking town in America, the owner is less likely to receive objections where monolingualism is common. The fact that the restaurant owner uses a British English dialect in America is another matter. The British owner may be embraced in the community where they think that British English is more proper than American English – based on such naïve beliefs as that Americans tend to sloppily contract their words and use too much slang. The opposite can be true if the community feels linguistically insecure about their form of language; they might mock the British owner for sounding too proper to them. But the Americans might not know if the owner's variety of English is on the high or low prestige end of the dialect spectrum in the UK. It would be ironic if the community feels threatened by what is a stigmatized form of English in Britain.

10.3.1 Language ideology about sign languages

Language ideology also shapes how we think and what we believe about sign languages. There are common misconceptions that are found around the world about sign languages: "it is all gestures," "it doesn't have a grammar," "its grammar is more flexible than spoken languages," "it is not a language because it doesn't have a writing system," "it is a broken visual form of spoken language," and "it is a universal language for Deaf people around the world." These misconceptions are based on the mistaken idea that sign languages cannot be real language. The common belief is that language is to be spoken; communication that is not by speech is not language. This belief is simply unfounded based on the evidence about sign languages. Despite this fact, it is difficult to make a dent in some people's language ideology of "language equals speech" because it is all they have known.

For example, during the 20th century in the United States, English-only and anti-immigration sentiments ran high and assimilation was the goal. This further informed the belief of educators and administrators serving students with hearing loss that ASL was linguistically inferior to English because of the differences in structure and vocabulary. Deaf students in schools were discouraged from signing because it marked them as different. Instead, they were trained to use speech in order to appear as "normal" or "civilized" as possible. From that time, educators' and administrators' language ideology maintained (and has continued maintaining) the belief that ASL is a "broken" or "improper" form of English with missing morphological and grammatical elements. Such a view sees the grammatical differences between ASL and English and interprets them as showing that ASL fails as a visual representation of English. As indicated in the previous chapters on the grammar of sign languages, ASL does not fail as a linguistic system; it is as valid as any natural language in its structure, vocabulary, and language practices and it does not need to be corrected simply because it is a different language in a different modality from English.

Unfortunately, it is not only ASL that faces such misconceptions. There are many sign languages that suffer the same fate. In Italy, a signed system, Signed Italian *italiano segnato*, was created to accommodate the structure of spoken Italian even though Italian Sign Language (Lingua dei Segni Italiana (LIS)) is perfectly fine as a natural language with its own structure. In Belgium, there are five different dialects of Flemish Sign Language (Vlaamse Gebarentaal (VGT)) but Signed Dutch was developed as a preferred alternative to those dialects because it followed Dutch grammar and was considered to be a proper language. The preference for spoken languages over sign languages is global, especially in the context of education, where people are not informed, or in some cases convinced, of the linguistic structure of sign language. Such preference is the proverbial tip of the iceberg, that is, language ideology influencing language practice and status.

10.4 Language management

Language management includes efforts to intervene in or plan how language forms should be used, promoted, changed, or prohibited. For example, in the previous section when we discussed the hypothetical restaurant owner, you can see how we avoided using gendered pronouns when referring to the owner. Before we pointed that out, what was your default assumption about the gender of that owner? Was it a man? A woman? A nonbinary person? What made you think of that person's gender? Was it in the language we wrote or was it based on your worldview? Gender is a socially constructed dichotomy that divides people based on biological sex traits, but the concepts of gender are not same for every community in the world. If a cisgender owner had been identified, we could use an appropriately gendered pronoun such as "he" or "she," as commonly practiced in our community. If that owner identified as transgender or nonbinary, we could use their preferred pronouns out of respect for the owner: "he, him, his, and himself"; "she, her, hers, and herself"; "they, them, their, and themselves"; "xe, xem, xyr, and xemself"; "ve, ver, vis, and verself"; "per, pers, perself"; or even no pronoun at all. For someone who is comfortable practicing preferred pronoun conventions, this won't be a problem, but for someone who is not, it can be a potential conflict.

So what can we do about it? We could propose one pronoun system that is not based on gender and everyone, be they cisgender, transgender, or nonbinary, could use the genderless pronouns to refer to each other. If the system were adopted, we would have to plan it in a way that would become part of our institutions and therefore our reality. But of course, with any change comes resistance from people who want to keep everything as it is. Proposing, implementing, and monitoring language patterns such as these falls under the domain of language management. Such language planning or intervention can be categorized into three different types: status planning, corpus planning, and acquisition planning. Attitude planning is another type but it often overlaps with the other types; it concerns the goal of changing people's attitudes toward a particular language or dialect and promoting monolingualism or multilingualism.

10.4.1 Status planning

There are two types of language status: (1) the development and existence of a language and (2) the official recognition of a language in legislation. Status planning concerns the latter type of language status; it involves political strategies in raising or lowering the status of a language. Considering how powerful and intractable the negative language ideology against sign languages is, it is easy to see why such official language recognition is necessary in order to gain language rights.

In the case of Italy, LIS has not been formally recognized as an official language of the Italian Deaf community, but there is an ongoing effort to make that happen so the language right of Italian Deaf people can be preserved. In 1999, a law was passed to protect and preserve the diversity of languages but somehow LIS was not part of it. The reason is that the law only considers historical languages, national language from other countries, and regional dialects, all of them spoken in local communities that exist in different regions. A group of Italian Deaf people is not formally recognized as a community because they are scattered all over the country. This law secures funding for those linguistic minorities to exercise their civil rights and to conduct language policy and planning efforts. The Italian Deaf community cannot assert their language rights under this law. The only legal provisions that offer limited protection of LIS are disability laws, but they are not enough to promote the linguistic civil rights of Deaf people and reduce barriers in order to have full participation in the society. In 2005, a petition was filed with the Italian Parliament to get them to recognize LIS as an official language. Seven years later, the LIS recognition bill had been approved by one house of the Italian Parliament, *la Camera del Senato*, and was passed on to another house, *la Camera dei Deputati*, to discuss the bill. It was an exciting moment for the Italian Deaf community, but then inexplicably, LIS was replaced by a new name, "linguaggio o tecnica comunicativa mimico-gestuale," which is translated as "mimed-gestural language or communication technique." This implied that LIS was merely a system of gestures; this goes against decades of linguistic research that points to the linguistic system of LIS. As of this date, the fight to have LIS recognized as a language in the legislation continues.

Brazil was in a similar situation as Italy until it passed the Brazilian Sign Language (Lingua Brasileira de Sinais) law, commonly referred as the Libras law, in 2002. Such a law was necessary because although there is a general belief that Brazil is a homogeneous society with one language, that directly contradicts the multilingual and multicultural reality, with over 200 languages used in the country. Before legal protections, it was very difficult for the Brazilian Deaf community to assert their civil rights with access to public infrastructure using Libras. Under the Libras law, sign language interpreting is available on TV, schools permit the use of Libras, and universities provide sign language and interpreting training courses. This is not to say that the Deaf community finally has complete participation in the society. The struggles still exist in some areas of public life and the Deaf community will have to continue to advocate for their needs as a cultural and linguistic minority.

The United States is in a different legal context. The American Deaf community can assert their civil rights including communication access, but it is not under any language law; it is disability law, including the Americans with Disability Act of 1990, that recognizes such rights. Under this federal law, discrimination in employment, public services, public accommodations, and telecommunications on the basis of disability is prohibited. Based on hearing disability, Deaf people have rights to communication access in any manner including sign language interpreting; but it is important to remember that this does not mean that ASL is legally recognized. If the American Deaf community wants to have ASL officially recognized by the United States, it will only lead to complications because of two major factors. First, the United States has a governmental structure in which the federal government shares sovereignty with state governments, leading to the reality that states deal with language recognition on their own. Second, at the federal level there are no official languages – not even English has been recognized as an official language. Although the country is a multilingual nation with a complicated history of discrimination and oppression against those with limited privileges, any movement toward official language policy could very well lead to an English-only ruling. Attempts at legal recognition of ASL and other non-English languages would have such an alternative outcome to consider. To date, some US states do recognize ASL in their legislation, but it is typically in the education and interpreting contexts as a language of the Deaf community, rarely as a language right that needs to be protected.

10.4.2 Corpus planning

Corpus planning often happens in conjunction with status planning with the effort to standardize, modify, revitalize, or purify a language. Corpus planning is different from building a description-based corpus, which is a collection of representative samples of a language; the purpose of this latter sort of language corpus is to recognize and verify the actual language use and variation in a language. While corpus building can be part of corpus planning, the purpose of corpus building is different from the purpose of corpus planning. Corpus planning is a form of intervention that may preserve or change a language. The activities of corpus planning include creating or modifying writing systems, coining new words or expressions, expanding vocabulary, controlling or limiting language borrowing, publishing a dictionary, preparing language materials, and standardizing a language. In Brazil, with the passage of the Libras law, the Brazilian Deaf community and their advocates and allies were able to organize in various ways, including developing Libras courses and interpreter training programs at universities. These programs require educational materials about the structure and use of Libras, including a sign language textbook, dictionary, and videos. The production of such resources requires a collaborative corpus planning effort with different stakeholders, and has resulted in tremendous progress for sign language and the Deaf community in Brazil.

However, working on such recognition and standards can be political at times, as has been seen in the case of ASL. During the 19th century, American educators already had the right idea when they decided to use a natural sign language as the most effective instructional medium to support Deaf students' learning. The clear advantage of using a sign language is that it was immediately accessible for the students. Furthermore, students could socialize with each other using the language. Unfortunately, the opponents of sign language had a different idea. They thought that compared to English, sign language made Deaf students look primitive, and this hindered them from integrating into the mainstream society. With the sign language ban in 1880 (described in Chapter 8), Deaf children in America (and around the world) were deprived of sign language as the source of their critical development. The "language equals speech" ideology of the time further reduced the status of sign language. A breakthrough came in the 1960s, when linguistic researchers, William C. Stokoe and his Deaf associates, Carl Croneberg and Dorothy Casterline, recognized the linguistic structure of the sign language used by Deaf Americans. After completing their linguistic analysis, they released their linguistic dictionary of sign language with the entries organized according to properties of ASL, using special symbols for handshapes; crucially, they also gave the language they were working on a new name, *American Sign Language* (ASL). Prior to that, it was simply called "sign language." This should have been a moment of celebration for the signing community, but instead it was a moment of confusion, anxiety, and anger. Many had thought English was the language they used, not ASL. Recognition of ASL as distinct from English was the peak moment of linguistic insecurity for signers who had been indoctrinated with the belief that English was superior to ASL.

In 1988, a movement gave a huge push to the ideological shift from "language equals speech" to "language is language," and that movement was known as Deaf President Now (DPN). The DPN protest at Gallaudet University (then Gallaudet College) gained national attention to the issue of sign language use and Deaf culture, because the university board failed to pick a Deaf candidate over a hearing candidate to lead as the college's next president. There had been no history of a Deaf person leading the university as president since 1864. The week-long protest resulted in the resignation of the hearing president and the appointment of the first Deaf president. Within two years, the American with Disabilities Act of 1990 was passed and opened doors for Deaf people to exercise their language right at some levels. The publication of the ASL linguistic dictionary and the naming of sign language were arguably a historical precedent that gave way to intentional corpus planning in the following decades. Due to the ideological and linguistic shift, ASL is now one of the more popular languages in foreign language programs in K-12 and postsecondary educational institutions in the United States. The scientific and humanistic studies of ASL have grown into the respectable fields of sign language linguistics, interpreting, and Deaf Studies. With the growing demand, ASL instruction is a multimillion dollar industry with teacher training programs, interpreting programs, teaching and interpreting certification bodies, language proficiency assessments, language textbooks, dictionaries, media, online materials, and entertainment. All of these can be categorized as part of corpus planning.

Language standardization is another corpus planning process by which people establish and maintain standard language forms. It includes a selection of one language variety over others, a promotion or enforcement of one variety by authority, an elaboration of one variety including vocabulary expansion and planned structure, and a codification of a variety to maximize linguistic functions. There are two types of standardization: a process that is imposed from an authority figure or body and a process that is natural and spontaneous within a community. The first type is exemplified by the case of the Sign Language of Netherlands (Nederlandse Gebarentaal, NGT) where the standardization of NGT was done as a direct response to the Dutch government's 1996 report. The condition was that if the Deaf Dutch community wanted to have NGT legally recognized as an official language of the community, NGT must be standardized for use in schools. This stirred a controversy in the community because NGT was already a full-fledged language, so standardization was not a linguistic condition; it was a political condition that placed the educational need for standardization over the natural variation in the community. Over the objection of some Deaf people and linguistic researchers, the standardization project was headed by a group of linguists, native Deaf signers, and native hearing signers to cover three different areas: language planning and education, selection of signs (for dictionaries), and lexicographical procedures. Despite the overall success of the project with the dictionary database, the government has not fulfilled its promise to officially recognize NGT on the basis of language standardization.

The second type of standardization is a natural spontaneous process within a community with their adoption of and preference for different variants. For example, in the 1990s, the Flemish Deaf community went through the process to get their language, VGT, recognized by the Flemish government in Belgium. VGT has five different dialects that are bound to five different regions with their own deaf schools. As with the Dutch government, one condition on recognition was to have VGT standardized for educational purposes including language classes. In 1997, the Flemish Deaf community strongly rejected this kind of imposed standardization, out of concern that history would repeat itself. Toward the end of the 1970s, one deaf school decided to promote a signed Dutch system instead of VGT as a medium of instruction because the signed Dutch system was aligned with spoken Dutch as a way to achieve lexical unification across Belgium. Signed Dutch was designed as a convenient communication tool to serve the needs of hearing people rather than for Deaf people. This resulted in linguistic insecurity within the VGT community since Dutch was the standard language for the country and the community thought it was impossible for VGT to be prestigious. But during the 1990s, the Deaf community learned about the linguistic aspects of VGT through workshops and courses and this led them to reject Signed Dutch and embrace VGT as their natural language. Even with the variation within VGT, they were able to adopt multiple variants through various forms of contact including travel, use of webcams, and meetings, and the community let the variants work themselves out by community preference, geographic boundaries, and media exposure.

10.4.3 Acquisition planning

Language development is a crucial component of a child's life. The period during which language development typically takes place also features a great deal of social and emotional development. Resources have been developed and committed to support parents' interactions with children and teachers' instructional methods for students. However, a lot depends on how Deaf students' language and communication needs are ideologically framed. The choice of ideological frame determines the choices made in language acquisition planning, including the medium of instruction, the manner of teaching literacy, the number of languages used, and preparation and certification programs for professionals in education.

One frame is that hearing loss is generally seen as a communication disorder, and thus Deaf people are perceived to be in need of serious intervention with listening and speech therapy.

Such a view can include what is considered "support" from signs, or it can completely reject the use of signs. The communication disorder frame has been in existence since 1880 (and longer before that) when the language-based exclusion policy was instituted in Milan, Italy, and promoted to the rest of the world. There have indeed been cases where Deaf people are able to acquire the spoken language of their community after undergoing speech and listening therapy. The extent of the financial, mental, and social cost to make such therapy effective varies greatly for different Deaf people. Importantly, there are many Deaf children who don't directly benefit from speech training, even with the recent improvements in hearing assistive technology. The longer children have to go without having full access to language, the more serious is the resulting language deprivation as a medical trauma.

Prior to the 1960s, Deaf students in the United States were subjected to a language policy that excluded ASL as the medium of education and enforced English instruction instead. The language ideology shared by educators and students alike was that English was the only "language" and signing was a broken form of English. Because of that ideology, English-based sign codes were created as an intervention to support Deaf students' English development in the 1960s and 1970s. English-based sign codes were largely preferred in specialized educational programs for Deaf students, which maintained the language ideology that English was the norm. Signs were initialized to match the first initials of English words and arranged in English word order. That reinforced the belief that signing must follow English. This theme has been repeated in the history of many sign languages taught in schools, including VGT, LIS, and LSF as discussed in this chapter.

As for hearing assistive technology, the use of hearing aids and cochlear implants is very common now in the Deaf community. Deaf people who wear hearing aids and cochlear implants do receive benefits of hearing to different degrees. Cochlear implant technology has improved tremendously over the past years. There are reports of people who were implanted at a young age who can now communicate by speech without relying on any visual cues. However, the spoken language outcomes even for children who receive their implants early are quite variable, and some are not able to exclusively rely on spoken language. This problem is largely related to the widely held language ideology that speech is the default form of language. The medical and educational institutions are often connected ideologically in supporting Deaf children's spoken language development, so medical and educational professionals continue to perpetuate the mistaken ideology that sign language is harmful to Deaf children's communication development. Families, schools, and medical establishments that continue to avoid using sign language may contribute to language deprivation as a form of trauma for Deaf people, especially those who don't benefit from hearing aids or cochlear implants. The language-based exclusion policy is one example of acquisition planning that promotes either the educational method of speaking and listening or the sign-supported speech method, which emphasizes speech acquisition and development including some vocabulary items used in sign.

The other frame is the promotion of Deaf students' right to have a sign language as their first natural language for the sake of communication access as well as cognitive and social development. A recent educational shift is the growth of bilingual and bicultural (BiBi) education programs for Deaf students that use a sign language as one of their options. The BiBi approach is based on the educational philosophy that students' proficiency in their first language should be fostered in order to stimulate cognitive processes in language acquisition; with the foundation of the first language and the promotion of bilingualism in school, students can function just as well in the second language. As you recall, the vast majority of Deaf children are born to hearing families whose home language is typically spoken, so BiBi educational programs are a common setting for Deaf students' sign language acquisition and development.

However, not every school adopts the BiBi approach; there are many schools that only provide oral communication services with hearing assistive devices to support spoken communication development in students with hearing loss. In the United States, federal laws mandate educational accommodations and specialized services for children with disabilities, including Deaf students (Section 504 of the Rehabilitation Act of 1973 (504 Plans), the Americans with Disability Act of 1990, and the Individuals with Disabilities Education Act (IDEA)). Nonetheless, the laws are either interpreted differently or minimally enforced in some schools, resulting in inconsistency in language and communication support services. Coupling this enforcement problem with the spoken language ideology in medical establishments, language deprivation is a real risk for Deaf children with limited access to language during the age period of zero to three years, which is a critical period of language development.

In the 2000s, there has been a movement in the United States to advocate for Deaf kindergarteners to have access to both ASL and English. The national campaign Language Equality and Acquisition for Deaf Kids (LEAD-K) is the latest effort along this line. It starts at the state level, recognizes the problems with early intervention programs that are exclusively auditory-based, and puts the spotlight on the injustice of denying Deaf children's exposure to sign language. The national campaign aims to raise public awareness about Deaf children's sense-based communication and language needs and to change public policy on the education of Deaf children. As recently as 2016, a Deaf white American male, Nyle DiMarco, has gained fame as a winner of the 22nd cycle of *America's Next Top Model* and the 22nd season of *Dancing with the Stars*. He's a fourth-generation member of a Deaf family whose home language is ASL. Instead of sitting back and enjoying the national fame, he has become a spokesperson for LEAD-K and used his fame as a platform to put a spotlight on the problem of language deprivation under which Deaf children continue to suffer as a result of language-based exclusion policies. This is, by far, the largest platform that a Deaf activist like DiMarco has successfully commanded with the goal of ending the epidemic of language deprivation and promoting the use of ASL and English as the human right of Deaf children. The promotion of BiBi educational approaches and the LEAD-K initiative are examples of acquisition planning that promotes the use of sign language in schools.

As with any corpus planning effort, there are bound to be challenges in implementing a policy that goes against the mainstream ideology about language. To LEAD-K and DiMarco's activism, there has been a pushback from people and organizations who support listening and spoken language (LSL) therapy and auditory verbal therapy (AVT) with hearing assistive devices on social and mass media. The common refrain in their rebukes is this: "Speaking deaf [sic] people are not language deprived." While ASL enjoys its status as one of the popular foreign languages in K-12 and postsecondary settings, the benefit of learning ASL extends more to hearing people than for Deaf people. For example, while parents are encouraged to use baby signs with their hearing infants to support their communication development, parents of deaf infants are usually discouraged by medical establishments from using signs lest it hurt the children's speech and hearing development, so the language ideology and coercion restricts ASL access. The number of deaf schools with specialized services for signing Deaf children has been reduced, so access to ASL is becoming restricted. Deaf people still have trouble securing ASL interpretation services in some places. Deaf people feel isolated in their own non-signing families who don't enforce ASL in their own home. The intersection of language ideology and disability oppression paints reality for Deaf people differently than for hearing people, and it takes time, energy, and resources for corpus planning to overcome such ideology and oppression.

10.5 Conclusion

Language practices, language ideologies, and language management are aspects of language policy that can be explicit, implicit, or hidden. For sign language communities, an explicit language policy is desirable for protection against the ideological hegemony of standard language and the deficit view of disability that subjects Deaf people to auditory-based intervention instead of cultural intervention with existing sign languages. We have seen that advocates and allies in sign language communities have engaged in different forms of planning, including status planning, corpus planning, and acquisition planning to establish a federal law to protect language rights and to implement programs and activities to preserve and spread languages. Despite such legal protections, there is an ideological threat against the use of sign language in education as a language right.

For this reason, the World Federation of the Deaf (WFD), the international nonprofit and nongovernmental organization of Deaf associations, followed the United Nations' Convention on the Rights of Persons with Disabilities (CRPD) with its own statement that highlights the local and global threats against sign language communities as cultural and linguistic minorities. The WFD has issued signed translation videos of the CRPD in several sign languages, including those from Australia, Belgium, Canada, Denmark, Germany, Portugal, Sweden, Russia, and Serbia. It is important to provide such accessibility to the CRPD because it contains language that requires states to recognize human and language rights of Deaf people, recognize and promote the use of sign languages, and to support bilingual education for Deaf people. With the right partners, legal tools, and compassion, sign language communities can advance with their demand for language recognition and protection as a basic human right.

Discussion questions

1   What are the three components of language policy and planning and how are they different from each other?
2   What do Signed English, Signed Dutch, and Signed Italian have in common? What purpose do such systems serve?
3   The majority of Deaf people are born to hearing families whose primary language is not a sign language. Often, the hearing families are at loss when they are dealing with Deaf children's communication needs. As a BiBi advocate who is involved in sign language acquisition planning, what resources and services would you recommend to fulfill the communication needs of their children in order to lessen the effect of language deprivation?

Further reading

Adam, R. (2015). Standardization of sign languages. *Sign Language Studies*, *15*(4), 432–445.
This article provides an overview of sign language standardization that occurred in different countries.

Eichmann, H. (2009). Planning sign languages: Promoting hearing hegemony? Conceptualizing sign language standardization. *Current Issues in Language Planning*, *10*(3), 293–307.
This article discusses the primacy of hearing people in sign language standardization and frames it as a problem for Deaf communities.

Humphries, T., Kushalnagar, P., Mathur, G., Napoli, D. J., Padden, C., Rathmann, C., & Smith, S. R. (2012). Language acquisition for deaf children: reducing the harms of zero tolerance to the use of alternative approaches. *Harm Reduction Journal, 9*, 16.
This article discusses language deprivation as an actual harm to Deaf children and presents different solutions to reduce the harm.

Meulder, M. D. (2015). The legal recognition of sign languages. *Sign Language Studies, 15*(4), 498–506.
This article provides an overview of the different types of legal recognition of sign languages.

Reagan, T. G. (2010). *Language policy and planning for sign languages.* Washington, DC: Gallaudet University Press.
This book contains a general overview on language policy and planning, with the main focus on American Sign Language and its history.

Bibliography

7 September 2016: WFD position paper on the language rights of deaf children. (2016, November 18). Retrieved from https://wfdeaf.org/news/resources/wfd-position-paper-on-the-language-rights-of-deaf-children-7-september-2016/

Behares, L. E., Brovetto, C., & Crespi, L. P. (2012). Language policies in Uruguay and Uruguayan Sign Language (LSU). *Sign Language Studies, 12*(4), 519–542, 627–628.

Geraci, C. (2012). Language policy and planning: the case of Italian Sign Language. *Sign Language Studies; Washington, 12*(4), 494–518, 626–627.

Hall, W. C. (2017). What you don't know can hurt you: the risk of language deprivation by impairing sign language development in deaf children. *Maternal and Child Health Journal; New York, 21*(5), 961–965.

Johnson, R. E., Liddell, S., & Erting, C. (1989). Unlocking the curriculum: principles for achieving access in deaf education. Working Paper 89–3. *Graduate Studies and Research.*

Krausneker, V. (2015). Ideologies and attitudes toward sign languages: an approximation. *Sign Language Studies, 15*(4), 411.

Nakamura, K. (2006). Creating and contesting signs in contemporary Japan: language ideologies, identity, and community in flux. *Sign Language Studies; Washington, 7*(1), 11–29,102.

Quadros, R. M. de (2012). Linguistic policies, linguistic planning, and Brazilian Sign Language in Brazil. *Sign Language Studies; Washington, 12*(4), 543–564, 628–629.

Quer, J., & Quadros, R. M. de. (2015). Language policy and planning in deaf communities. In A. C. Schembri & C. Lucas (Eds.), *Sociolinguistics and deaf communities* (pp. 120–145). Cambridge, England: Cambridge University Press.

Schermer, T. (2012). Sign language planning in the Netherlands between 1980 and 2010. *Sign Language Studies, 12*(4), 467–493.

Spolsky, B. (2004). *Language policy.* Cambridge, England: Cambridge University Press.

Van Herreweghe, M., & Vermeerbergen, M. (2009). Flemish Sign Language standardisation. *Current Issues in Language Planning, 10*(3), 308–326.

Chapter 11

Conclusion

This book is primarily about natural sign languages, the languages of Deaf communities that naturally emerge when signers are together. We focused on American Sign Language (ASL), the language used in the United States and most parts of Canada. Our goal was to provide an overview of the variants of ASL that are used by Deaf community members with different backgrounds, noting those features that might be related to particular types of signing or signers.

The book summarized sign language research in a number of areas. First, we showed what research has said about the grammatical structure of ASL and other sign languages. We showed that signs have parts, and the organization and patterning of these parts can be analyzed using the same abstract phonological principles as those used for analyzing spoken languages, although the use of the visual/manual modality means that sign languages are different from spoken languages in particular ways. We raised the question of whether sign languages have syllables; syllables are units that organize the structure of words rhythmically, and many phonological principles are based on syllabic units. We also looked at prosodic structure in sign languages, and saw that various nonmanual elements form important components of sign language prosody.

In the areas of morphology and syntax, we found again many similarities to the organizing principles of spoken languages, with some important modality effects. We discussed implicit rules for the formation of words and sentences. We saw that ASL has several devices for creating new words, including a particularly productive process of compounding. We found that ASL has morphological processes that apply to verbs, but unlike English they do not mark tense, instead showing person or location agreement and aspect. ASL also has a productive process for forming complex classifier predicates, which include an obligatory depictive component. While the neutral, basic word order of sentences in ASL is Subject–Verb–Object, this order can be changed through various processes, including one that places a sentential topic in the sentence-initial position. Nonmanual marking is crucial for topics and questions, including polar (yes/no) questions and wh-questions. Wh-questions allow for the placement of a wh-word in a variety of sentential positions; it can be at the beginning or end of a sentence or in both positions, or it can occur in its sentence-internal *in situ* position. We also saw that ASL displays very specific patterns for marking negation with different negative signs, and that the placement of a negative sign has great consequences for the interpretation of a sentence.

Following our set of chapters on the grammar of ASL, we turned our attention to how sign languages are acquired in different contexts. We started with the context providing the most accessible input: Deaf children whose Deaf, signing parents use ASL with them from the day that they are born. Such children have early access to fluent signers, and their language development follows much the same path as that of hearing children acquiring a spoken language from their parents. However, most Deaf people do not learn a sign language this way. In a small proportion, input is provided from birth by parents who are themselves late learners and therefore some inconsistencies can be expected. Much more often, the Deaf child's hearing parents do not know a sign language at all, or might be learning it together with their children. In this context, children's initial access to ASL input is delayed, and the quality of their input may also be affected. While children are able to make up for some deficiencies or irregularities in their input, they must have input at an early age, and lifelong effects in competence and processing can be observed in those whose language acquisition is delayed.

For those who do not receive accessible input in a natural sign language, the child's own language drive will enable them to build a home sign system that has many of the characteristics of a natural language. Even in young children, sophisticated systems of gestural symbols arranged in a regular pattern can be self-created. If no natural sign language input is provided and the spoken language is not attained, home sign can be a Deaf person's means of communication into adulthood. We saw that adult homesign systems have remarkable complexity and sophistication, although they are not ideal communication systems for many reasons. They illustrate that humans are extremely well prepared for integration of language, but they also emphasize the essential need for a communicative community.

Finally, we turned our attention to consider signing communities in more detail. We saw that sign languages, as well as spoken languages, change and evolve over time and distance, and that such changes lead to differences between groups that can lead to a new variety, dialect, or language. Languages are used within a social milieu, and this context affects language use. In the case of ASL and other sign languages, formation of a Deaf community tends to be associated with educational programs for Deaf children, even when those programs do not include a sign language. Because of the role of social context in language, members of different communities have specific assumptions, values, and attitudes about language varieties. These are based on social factors, not strictly linguistic ones, since the linguistic view treats all languages on a par. Nevertheless the social perceptions are real and have forceful effects on languages and their users. Importantly, language users are generally members of more than one social group and they use language in multiple social domains. For signers, their membership in a Deaf community must be understood together with their membership in other communities, related to their racial and ethnic identity, their line of work, and all the other factors of their life. While we can and do study language structure independent of such factors, including them allows our study to be more explanatory and more holistic.

As we examined the relationship between languages and their contexts, we also were reminded that language use in these contexts is not accidental or random. There are explicit and implicit rules about how language is used in different contexts, and some of these are very specific to sign languages. As minority languages in a minority modality, sign languages may be in special need of explicit recognition and policy planning. This should not mean that others make the plans, of course; rather, Deaf signing community members themselves can set up expectations and work toward such goals with their allies.

While we covered a great deal of material in this small book, there is a lot of research on sign languages that has not even been mentioned. In addition to the areas discussed, there is now a growing and exciting field of sign language semantics, the study of how meanings are derived from words, sentences, and discourses. There is also a great deal of research on the psycholinguistics and neurolinguistics of sign languages. These studies investigate matters such as how signers access individual words in their mental lexicon, how signers put together sentences in real time, what the effects of factors such as frequency and iconicity are in language processing, what happens in the brain of signers when they access a sign language, how the neural structures for language are similar to and different from those used for spoken languages, and many more. And of course, even in the areas covered we were only able to summarize a fraction of the existing research. We encourage interested readers to look at the works listed in "Further reading" and "Bibliography" at the end of each chapter to see where we found the research we reported and some of the other kinds of research that exists.

There is much more still to be done, of course. In every area of study there are multiple open questions; probably there are more questions to be answered than answers already found. We are happy to play our own small roles in the work toward answering – and asking – more questions, and we hope that more researchers will join the cause in the years to come.

Index

Note: Italic page numbers denote figures and bold page numbers denote tables.

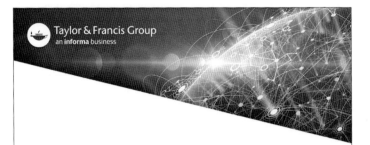